QM Library

23 1356206 5

D1639681

WITHDRAWN
FROM STOCK
QMUL LIBRARY

SEVENTH EDITION

The Scientific Basis of Oral Health Education

© 2014, British Dental Association

ISBN: 978-1-907923-07-4

All rights reserved. No part of this publication may be reproduced, stored in a retrieval
system, or transmitted in any form or by any means electronic, mechanical, photocopying,
recording or otherwise, without either the permission of the publishers or a licence
permitting restricted copying in the United Kingdom issued by the Copyright Licensing
Agency Ltd, Saffron House, 6-10 Kirby Street, London EC1N 8TS.

QM LIBRARY (WHITECHAPEL)

SEVENTH EDITION

The Scientific Basis of Oral Health Education

R S Levine OBE

Department of Oral Surgery
Leeds Dental Institute
University of Leeds
Leeds
LU2 9LU

C R Stillman-Lowe

Independent Oral Health Promotion Adviser
7 Broadwater Road
Twyford
Reading
RG10 0EX

First published in 1976; this edition published 2014.

Published by the British Dental Association
64 Wimpole Street, London, W1G 8YS

Contents

Preface

The first edition of *The Scientific Basis of Dental Health Education* appeared in 1976 and was a slim booklet with a green cover. It arose from a joint attempt by the British Association for the Study of Community Dentistry and the Health Education Council, who published it, to refine and standardise the advice given to the public and to ensure that such advice was scientifically sound. The need for this document grew from the problem of confusing and sometimes conflicting dental health education messages being provided by professional and commercial bodies. The strength of the original document was that it came from an independent and authoritative source and was based on a consensus of scientific opinion from a group of the leading dental experts of the day.

Over the intervening 38 years, the document has grown through five further editions to become one of the most widely used and accepted sources of information on oral health, both in the UK and abroad.

The scientific evidence on the causes and prevention of oral disease is constantly evolving and this new edition updates the evidence base for the range of topics previously covered. While primarily written for a UK readership, the use of previous editions in many other countries is recognised in this edition by the inclusion of information, evidence and opinion from international sources. To the four key messages given in the summary section, a fifth has been added on smoking cessation to highlight the importance of smoking as a risk factor for oral disease. Prominence is given to the concept of common risk factors that link oral disease with other non-communicable diseases and the section on behavioral change, central to the prevention of the main oral diseases, has been expanded. The chapter on periodontal disease has been extensively revised and includes a section on the association with obesity and diabetes, which together with smoking are now recognised as important risk factors.

The prevention of oral cancer, with its poor survival rate remains a priority for dental professionals and the oral cancer chapter has been updated and extended to include a section on the link between the human papilloma virus and oropharyngeal cancer. Finally the reference list has been updated and extended to reflect the latest scientific evidence and opinion. To keep the book within a reasonable length, however, it does not attempt to cover the full scope of oral health promotion: this is covered well by other textbooks, listed in the further reading section. In England Public Health England issues guidance on the prevention of oral disease to the dental team in the form a document – *Delivering better oral health: an evidence-based toolkit for prevention*[1], which gives a prescriptive guide to prevention in a primary care setting. This new edition of *The Scientific Basis of Oral Health Education* provides the information and evidence to underpin this guidance and care has been taken to ensure that the two documents are consistent.

As before, it is hoped that this new edition will be used both in the UK and abroad by dental schools, dental postgraduate deans and directors to help standardise undergraduate and postgraduate teaching and by dental care professionals, whose role within the dental team has developed significantly since 1976. Those involved in general healthcare, such as medical practitioners, school nurses, health visitors, midwives, dieticians and pharmacists also have a vital role to play in oral health promotion, and it is hoped that this publication will be of value to them. Oral health promotion staff in the Salaried Dental Service frequently provide training for people who can influence health in the wider community, such as teachers, child carers and peer educators and they can safely rely on the messages in this book as the basis for their programmes. Finally, it must be recognised that oral health education material is provided by a wide range of agencies, including government and professional bodies, charities, and commercial organisations in the form of both patient education material and for product promotion, much of which is of the highest standard. This too should conform to agreed expert opinion and it is hoped that this publication will be of assistance to these bodies.

Above all, this document is offered in the sincere belief that oral health education is one of our most important responsibilities and must be approached with the same dedication and professional quality standards that are applied to the operative treatment of disease. Only by offering the public consistent and soundly based advice can we hope that health education messages achieve their intended function of enabling individuals to control and improve their own health, as part of a comprehensive programme of national and local public health initiatives designed to tackle the determinants of poor health.

Acknowledgements

As with the previous editions, a considerable debt of gratitude is owed to the panel of expert advisers, including a number of new members as well as several who were involved in the earlier editions. They have been generous with their time and advice to help ensure that the document remains a consensus of expert opinion. We are grateful to all those who took the time and contributed to this consultation process, especially members of the Scientific Advisory Committee of the British Dental Association, Public Health England and the President of the British Society of Dental Hygiene and Therapy.

A guide to using this book

The aim of this book is to provide a sound basis for giving information and advice on the main aspects of oral health. The summary that follows gives a brief overview of the main oral diseases and some other oral conditions, together with five key messages. These key messages are a consensus of expert opinion and should form the basis of all oral health advice given to the public and other professionals.

Throughout this document, important statements are given at the beginning of each chapter in the form of key points. In order to indicate the level of supporting scientific evidence for each of these key points a simple scheme called Evidence Base is used:

- Evidence Base A: Statements supported by very strong evidence from pooled research data (meta-analysis) or systematic literature reviews.
- Evidence Base B: Statements supported by the majority of relevant research studies.
- Evidence Base C: Statements that cannot be supported by a substantial body of research evidence, but where there is a consensus of scientific and professional opinion to support the statement.

More detailed information on Evidence Base is given in Chapter 1, together with sections on health education and the nature of scientific evidence.

Chapters 2 to 12 cover the various diseases that can affect the teeth and mouth as a whole together with information on their causes and means of prevention, including advice for the under fives and older people.

Summary

The two most common oral diseases are tooth decay, dental caries and gum disease, properly known as periodontal disease. The principal cause of dental caries is the frequent consumption of sugars, mainly in confectionery, snack foods and soft drinks, acting on the layer of bacteria on the tooth surface, which we call plaque. The sugars are rapidly converted into acid by plaque bacteria and the build up of acid attacks the tooth surface causing a cavity and if untreated, destruction of the tooth with pain and possibly infection.

The common form of periodontal disease is caused by poor oral hygiene, allowing bacteria in the form of plaque to build up round the necks of the teeth. The toxins released from plaque cause inflammation of the gums, a condition known as gingivitis. The later stage of periodontitis develops when the supporting bone around the teeth becomes progressively destroyed, so that the teeth become loose and painful. Smoking is now recognized as an important risk factor, as is diabetes, especially if poorly controlled. Unlike tooth decay, which is usually a rapid process, periodontal disease can take many years to reach the stage where teeth become loose and may be lost.

Dental erosion, which causes wearing away of the surfaces of teeth appears to be an increasing problem. The cause is usually acid in the soft drinks and juices increasingly being consumed by children and young adults, 50% of whom are now affected to some degree. Erosion can also be caused by gastric regurgitation, as can occur in pregnancy, or due to conditions such as hiatus hernia or bulimia.

There are many other diseases that occur in the mouth and there are some conditions arising elsewhere in the body that can have a visible effect within the mouth, such as anaemia and HIV infection (AIDS). The most life-threatening oral disease is oral cancer. This condition is increasing in prevalence in many countries and in the UK it is now more common than cervical cancer with over 6,500 new cases each year, most being smoking or alcohol related. About half of these cases prove fatal, but early diagnosis greatly improves the chance of survival. Dental patients who wish to give up smoking should be offered appropriate support to do so. More information on smoking cessation is provided in Appendix 1.

Dental disease is not an inevitable part of life and research has shown that much can be prevented by changes in behaviour. Such changes require knowledge and skills for people to make healthy choices. These are influenced by social and economic pressures both on individuals and communities and may account for the persistence of high levels of dental caries in economically depressed communities.

To promote good oral health there are five key messages:

1. **Diet:** reduce the consumption and especially the frequency of intake of drinks, confectionery and foods with sugars.
    Evidence Base B (Chapters 2 & 3)

The consumption of sugars, both the frequency and the amount, is important in determining the rate of tooth decay. When sugars are consumed, they should be part of a meal rather than between meals. Snacks and drinks should be free of added sugars, whenever possible. The frequent consumption of acidic drinks (such as fruit juice, squashes or carbonated drinks) should be avoided to help prevent dental erosion.

2. **Toothbrushing:** clean the teeth thoroughly twice every day with a fluoride toothpaste.
    Evidence base A (Chapters 2 & 4)

Effective daily toothbrushing with a fluoride toothpaste containing at least 1,000 parts per million of fluoride is the best way of preventing both caries and periodontitis. Other oral hygiene aids such as interdental brushes are best used after they have been demonstrated by a dentist, therapist or hygienist. Thorough brushing of all tooth surfaces and gum margins twice every day is of more value than more frequent cursory brushing. A small soft-to-medium texture toothbrush should be used to allow all tooth surfaces and gum margins to be cleaned easily and comfortably. Effective toothbrushing with a fluoride toothpaste will help control caries provided that the diet is favourable.

3. **Fluoride:** fluoridation of the water supply is a safe and effective public health measure.
    Evidence base A (Chapter 2)

Water fluoridation should be targeted at communities with higher caries levels. Where it is not feasible other fluoride strategies should be employed, such as community and school-based programmes to promote the use of fluoride toothpaste.

4. **Dental attendance:** have an oral examination every year.
    Evidence base C (Chapter 11)

Everyone, irrespective of age and dental condition, should have regular oral examinations at intervals of no more than 12 months for those under 18 years of age and no more than 24 months for all adults, so that cases of oral cancer or other oral diseases can be detected early and treated. This advice also applies to those without any natural teeth. Children and those at risk from oral disease, including smokers, may need to be seen more frequently, as advised by the dentist.

5. **Smoking:** encourage smoking cessation.
    Evidence base A (Chapters 4, 7 & Appendix 1)

Periodontal disease and oral cancers, as well as a wide range of chronic diseases, are strongly linked to smoking. It is an important role of the dental team to tell smokers of the risks from smoking and to assist them with smoking cessation by referring them to specialist local stop smoking services.

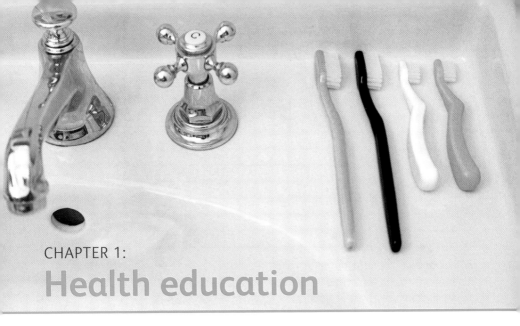

CHAPTER 1:
Health education

Key points

- Health education includes giving people personally relevant information about their health, which is based on a consensus of scientific evidence and opinion.
  Evidence Base C

- Health education programmes should be based on the best available evidence of what works and interventions should be evaluated in order to strengthen the evidence-base and improve the quality of health education.
  Evidence Base C

What is health education?

There are many definitions of health education, however one of the most useful is an adaptation of a definition from the World Health Organisation, "Health education is the process by which people are given information to enable them to exercise a greater degree of control over their own health".

The process of formulating and delivering health education messages includes a series of steps:

- The first step is to gain an understanding of the basic cause of the disease process under consideration. Taking dental caries as an example, the basic mechanism is the conversion of sugars in the diet into acid by the bacteria in plaque on the surfaces of the teeth.

- Next it is necessary to identify the essential causative factors. Some of these will be beyond individual personal control, such as environmental factors and genetics. However, others factors may be under the control of the individual and amenable to change. In the case of caries, factors under personal control can include the effective use of fluoride toothpaste and reducing the frequency of consumption of sugar-containing foods, drinks and confectionery.

- The third stage is to agree scientifically based and socially acceptable messages for the public aimed at encouraging beneficial behavioural changes. For the prevention of dental caries one could suggest that people should never consume sugars as part of their diet. However, compliance with this message is unrealistic because sugars are present in many foods and drinks, either naturally or added artificially. A more sensible message is "consume as little sugar as possible, especially avoiding sugars containing foods and drinks between meals and at bedtime". This message can reduce the risk from tooth decay and is more likely to be accepted, though it may need to be modified further where individuals' eating patterns do not conform to traditional mealtimes, and there may be no regular fixed bedtime for children.

- The final, and possibly the most difficult stage is that of communication. This process aims to ensure that key information is conveyed comprehensibly to the right target audience, in the right context, at the right time. In line with the World Health Organisation's Ottawa Charter[2], strategic aims for health promotion include traditional methods of health education, such as giving information and advice, thereby developing personal knowledge and skills. Health promotion may also include other elements: building public policies that support health; creating supportive environments; strengthening community action; and re-orientating health services. These are beyond the scope of this book, but health promotion, such as making the healthier choices easier, is vital if health education initiatives are to be successful.

The Common Risk Factor approach

There is a growing realisation that oral health is an integral part of overall health, and shares many common risk factors with leading chronic diseases, commonly referred to as non-communicable disease (NCDs)[3]. The World Health Assembly's resolution on oral health: action plan for promotion and integrated disease prevention urged Member States to adopt measures "to ensure that oral health is incorporated as appropriate into policies for the integrated prevention and treatment of chronic non-communicable disease and communicable disease, and into maternal and child health policies". Renal, oral and eye diseases pose a major health burden for many countries and these diseases have common risk factors and can benefit from common responses to NCDs. A meeting on Prevention and Control of NCDs concluded with a political declaration that commits governments of the world to significant and sustained action to address the rising burden of NCDs such as diabetes, cancers, cardiovascular and respiratory diseases, with oral diseases as an integral part. It is appropriate because the risk factors for oral diseases are common to other major chronic diseases. Therefore there is a need to incorporate programmes for promotion of oral health and prevention of oral diseases into programmes for the integrated prevention and treatment of all major NCDs. These programmes must be an integral part of the drive to reduce global health inequalities in both developed and developing countries[4].

Does health education and promotion work?

One of the most debated issues in public health is the effectiveness of health education and promotion. Health promotion extends health education beyond a focus on individual behaviour towards a wide range of social and environmental interventions. In many countries considerable resources are

QM LIBRARY (WHITECHAPEL)

spent on a range of interventions, ranging from one-to-one advice in primary care settings, to comprehensive healthy schools schemes, and mass media campaigns aimed for example at encouraging smoking cessation. The strength of the evidence-base for these interventions varies. A number of systematic reviews have examined studies in the dental field. Their findings were not always consistent, however the following conclusions were published in the report commissioned by Health Promotion Wales[5].

- There is clear evidence that oral health education/promotion can be effective in bringing about changes in people's knowledge, and in improving people's oral health.

- It is unclear whether one-off oral health promotion initiatives are sufficient to improve individuals' oral health significantly for long periods.

- There is evidence that programmes using more innovative approaches than the medical/behavioural model, have more potential for longer-term behaviour changes. They are more likely to be based on models of education and health behaviour that recognise the full variety of factors that influence a person's ability to comply with any messages given.

- Limited short-term behaviour changes are achievable using simple persuasive approaches. Greater or longer-term changes appear possible by using more tailored approaches that are based around active participation and addressing social, cultural and personal norms and values. The use of appropriate language and simple messages is important in avoiding confusion.

- Some studies show that health education which targets whole populations may increase inequalities in health.

- Preventive and comprehensive clinical approaches (including the appropriate use of fissure sealants) to oral health education can be effective in reducing the incidence of dental caries. However, this approach is intensive, and may not reach those in greatest need.

- Changing personal health behaviour appears to be more difficult for some groups than others; this may result in blaming the victim for not making the appropriate behaviour changes.

- Fluoride toothpaste is an important and effective method of delivering fluoride, although it will not reach the entire population. Evidence for the effectiveness of fluoride supplements, such as fluoride tablets, in home use and community schemes is lacking, especially for children using fluoride toothpastes on a regular basis.

The English Health Education Authority's review[6] concluded that:

- Oral health promotion, which includes the use of therapeutic agents incorporating fluoride, (whether in the form of toothpaste, tablets, drops, gels or rinses) is effective in reducing the development of caries. These improvements are cumulative and increase over time. Daily brushing with fluoride toothpaste is easier to achieve than regular use of other fluoride supplements. There is no evidence that oral health promotion per se affects caries rates, even if changes in behaviour are achieved, unless fluoride is being used.

- Clinical chairside advice and instruction aimed at improving oral hygiene have been demonstrated to be effective.

- Oral health education on an individual level aimed at improving oral hygiene is capable of reducing plaque levels. However, there is strong evidence that changes achieved are short-term and are not sustained. Interventions are effective even when very simple direct instruction is used. Cognitive-behavioural techniques are not required in order to achieve changes in plaque levels.

- The evidence suggests that oral health education is effective in increasing knowledge levels, but there is no evidence that changes in knowledge are causally related to changes in behaviour. However, there would appear to be an ethical responsibility for scientific knowledge to be disseminated to the public, irrespective of what the population does with that knowledge.

- Attempts to control individuals' consumption of sweet foods and drinks are generally not satisfactorily evaluated. However, when such interventions are directed at individuals, they appear to be of limited value.

In an age when cost-benefit assumes ever greater importance in healthcare, the effectiveness of oral health education in terms of the reduction in disease and healthcare costs is clearly of great significance, when investing scarce resources.

However, there is also an ethical obligation for health professionals possessing information that could reduce the prevalence of disease to inform the public accordingly, irrespective of whether a cost benefit can be proven to follow. The right of individuals to health education information was clearly defined by the Ottawa Charter in 1987[2]. Therefore, three things are clear. Firstly, that more research is needed with the aims of improving the quality of health education delivered and evaluating the results of interventions, including their sustainability. The second is that although strong evidence for the effectiveness of health education and promotion is lacking in some areas, this does not remove from health professionals the responsibility to provide the public with all available information for the promotion of good health. Finally, in order to be effective, health education needs to be properly planned, organised and evaluated, using the skills of the whole dental team, and the best quality and most appropriate resources.

Public health guidance on behaviour change

In 2014, the UK National Institute for Health and Care Excellence (NICE) published guidance on individual approaches to behaviour change[7]. The recommendations relevant to oral health education were as follows:

Recommendation 1

Develop a local behaviour change policy and strategy

National and local policy makers and commissioners of behaviour change services and their partners (see *Who should take action?*) should:

- Ensure policies and strategies aim to improve everyone's health and wellbeing.

- Use health equity audit to ensure health inequalities will not increase, and if possible will decrease as a result of the local behaviour change strategy and related programmes and interventions. (See NICE's local government briefing on health inequalities and population health for information about health equity audit).

- Develop a commissioning strategy, linked to relevant policies, for an evidence-based behaviour change programme of population, community, organisational and individual-level behaviour change interventions. For example, see NICE guidance on alcohol and obesity.

- Also note that Behaviour change: the principles for effective interventions (NICE public health guidance 6, 2007) recommends delivering individual interventions in tandem with complementary activities at the population, community and organisational levels.

- Work with the local community to develop the strategy (see Community engagement, NICE public health guidance 9).

- Ensure the strategy, and any related policies, are sustainable and meet local needs, identified through joint strategic needs assessments (JSNAs) and other local data.

- Identify the behaviours the strategy will address, and the outcomes it aims to achieve. Bear in mind that some interventions and programmes can address more than one behaviour (for example, sexual behaviour and alcohol consumption).

- Ensure the content, scale and intensity of each intervention is proportionate to the level of social, economic or environmental disadvantage someone faces and the support they need (proportionate universalism).
- Identify a leader within each local authority area, for example, the director of public health or an elected member of cabinet, to address specific behaviours (such as smoking and physical activity).

Recommendation 2

Ensure organisation policies, strategies, resources and training all support behaviour change

- Directors in national and local organisations whose employees deliver behaviour change interventions should ensure policies, strategies and resources are in place to provide behaviour change support for staff, as well as service users. This support could take the form of behaviour change services for staff. Or it could involve creating environments that support health-promoting behaviour (for examples, see NICE guidance on smoking and physical activity).

- National and local organisations whose employees deliver behaviour change interventions should review job descriptions and person specifications to check that they include behaviour change knowledge and skills (or competencies), if they are a specific part of someone's job (see recommendation 9).

- Managers of health, wellbeing and social care services should determine which staff in contact with the public are best placed to deliver different levels of a behaviour change intervention (see recommendation 9). They should ensure those staff have the knowledge and skills (or competencies) needed to assess behaviours and individual needs (see recommendation 8) and to deliver the intervention.

- Employers should ensure staff are aware of the importance of being supportive, motivating people and showing them empathy (see recommendation 12).

- Directors and managers should ensure staff receive behaviour change training and supervision related to their roles and responsibilities (see recommendation 9). They should also be offered on going professional development on behaviour change theories, methods and skills (see recommendation 12).

- Mentors and supervisors with relevant training and experience (see recommendations 11 and 12) should support staff who are delivering behaviour change interventions. This includes helping them to set their own goals, providing constructive feedback on their practice and encouraging them to be aware of their duty of care. It also involves making them aware of the likely perceptions and expectations of those taking part in behaviour change interventions and programmes.

Recommendation 3

Commission interventions from services willing to share intervention details and data

Commissioners of behaviour change services and their partners (see *Who should take action?*) should:

- Only commission behaviour change interventions and programmes that meet the recommendations in this guidance and in Behaviour change: the principles for effective interventions (NICE public health guidance 6).

- Ensure behaviour change interventions aim to both initiate and maintain change. Interventions should include techniques to address relapse and recognise that it is common.

- Commission interventions that are proven to be effective at changing and maintaining behaviour change. (See recommendation 4; also see NICE guidance on alcohol, diet, physical activity, sexual behaviour and smoking.)

- Specify in service specifications that providers:

  - make a detailed description of the intervention publicly available (see recommendation 6)

  - collate accurate, standardised and comparable routine data on behaviours that affect health and wellbeing. (For example, behaviours covered by the Public Health Outcomes Framework.)

- Commission interventions from providers who agree to make their evaluation and monitoring data available to commissioners and local and national organisations. (The aim is to aid the design, delivery and monitoring of service processes and outcomes.) **For example, data could be collected on:**

  - process assessment and quality assurance

  - health outcomes.

Recommendation 4

Commission high quality, effective behaviour change interventions

National and local policy makers, commissioners of behaviour change services and their partners (see *Who should take action?*) should:

- Find out whether behaviour change interventions and programmes that are already in place are effective, cost effective and apply evidence-based principles. (See Behaviour change: the principles for effective interventions, NICE public health guidance 6).
- Ensure that, when commissioning behaviour change interventions and programmes:
  - Evaluation plans tailored for the intervention and target behaviours are built in from the outset.
  - Resources (staff, time and funds) are allocated for independent evaluation of the short-, medium- and long-term outcomes.
  - A quality assurance process is in place to assess whether the intervention was delivered as planned (intervention fidelity), achieves the target behaviour change and health and wellbeing outcomes, and reduces health inequalities. (The frequency of quality assurance checks should be specified.)
  - There are quality assurance checks if an intervention has already been shown to be effective.
  - All information on intervention processes and outcomes is recorded in a form that can be made available if needed (for example, on a secure database).
- Commission and evaluate a pilot if it is not clear whether an intervention shown to be effective for a specific behaviour, population or setting can be applied to other behaviours, settings or populations (see recommendation 16).
- Commission an intervention for which there is no evidence of effectiveness only if it is accompanied by an adequately powered and controlled evaluation that measures relevant outcomes (see recommendation 16).
- Stop running interventions or programmes if there is good evidence to suggest they are not effective or are harmful.

Recommendation 5

Plan behaviour change interventions and programmes taking local needs into account

Commissioners and providers of behaviour change services, and intervention t designers (see *Who should take action?*) should:

- Work together and with other key stakeholders (for example, people who use services, communities and researchers) to select priority areas for interventions, based on local need.

- They should also identify suitable interventions that are acceptable to the target audiences.

- Take into account the local social and cultural contexts to ensure equitable access for everyone who needs help and make best use of existing resources and skills.

- Base behaviour change interventions and programmes on evidence of effectiveness (see recommendations 6 and 7).

- Take into account:

  - the objectives of the intervention or programme

  - evaluation plans (see recommendations 4 and 16)

  - the target population (including characteristics such as socioeconomic status)

  - whether there is a need to offer tailored interventions for specific subgroups (for example, see Preventing type 2 diabetes: risk identification and interventions for individuals at high risk, NICE public health guidance 38)

  - intervention characteristics: content, assessment of participants, mode of delivery, intensity and duration of the intervention, who will deliver it, where and when the training needs of those delivering the intervention or programme

  - the quality of the behavioural support provided by those delivering the intervention or programme availability of, and access to, services once the intervention has finished

  - follow up and support to maintain the new behaviour

  - plans to monitor and measure intervention fidelity.

Recommendation 6

Develop acceptable, practical and sustainable behaviour change interventions and programmes

Commissioners of behaviour change services and intervention designers (see *Who should take action?*) should:

- Work together and with other key stakeholders (for example, people who use services, communities and researchers) to develop (co-produce) behaviour change interventions and programmes that are acceptable, practical and sustainable. This should also reduce duplication between services.

- Develop interventions that:

  - are evidence-based

  - have clear objectives that have been developed and agreed with stakeholders

  - identify the core skills, knowledge and experience (competencies) needed to deliver the intervention (including for the specific behaviour change techniques used)

  - provide details of the training needed (including learning outcomes) for practitioners

  - include a monitoring and evaluation plan developed according to agreed objectives.

- Before implementing a behaviour-change intervention, describe in detail the principles it is based on. Put these details in a manual. This should include:

  - clearly stated objectives on what the intervention will deliver

  - the evidence base used (such as from NICE guidance on a specific topic)

  - an explanation of how the intervention works (mechanism of action), for example, by targeting capability, opportunity and motivation.

- Ensure manuals also include a detailed description of the intervention including:

  - resources, setting or context, activities, processes and outcomes (including a pictorial description of the relationship between these variables, such as a conceptual map or logic model)

- intervention characteristics (see recommendation 5)
- a clear definition of the behaviour change techniques used so that each component can be replicated (for example, by using a taxonomy)
- details of how to tailor the intervention to meet individual needs (see recommendation 8)
- plans to address long-term maintenance of behaviour change and relapse
- implementation details: who will deliver what, to whom, when and how.

- Make the manual publicly available, for example, on a website (provide copyright details and "training before use" requirements). If there are changes to an intervention during delivery, or after evaluation, ensure the manual is updated accordingly.

Recommendation 7

Use proven behaviour change techniques when designing interventions

Providers of behaviour change interventions and programmes and intervention designers should:

- Design behaviour change interventions to include techniques that have been shown to be effective at changing behaviour. These techniques are described in principle 4 of Behaviour change: the principles for effective interventions (NICE public health guidance 6) and include:

  - Goals and planning. Work with the client to:
    - agree goals for behaviour and the resulting outcomes
    - develop action plans and prioritise actions
    - develop coping plans to prevent and manage relapses
    - consider achievement of outcomes and further goals and plans.

  - Feedback and monitoring (for example, regular weight assessment for weight management interventions):
    - encourage and support self-monitoring of behaviour and its outcomes and
    - provide feedback on behaviour and its outcomes.

  - Social support. If appropriate advise on, and arrange for, friends, relatives, colleagues or 'buddies' to provide practical help, emotional support, praise or reward.

- Ensure the techniques used match the service user's needs (see recommendation 8).

- Consider using other evidence-based behaviour change techniques that may also be effective. See NICE guidance on alcohol, diet, physical activity, sexual behaviour and smoking for details of specific techniques.

- Clearly define and provide a rationale for all behaviour change techniques that have been included.

- Ensure novel techniques – or those for which the evidence base is limited – are evaluated (see recommendation 16).

- Consider delivering an intervention remotely (or providing remote follow-up) if there is evidence that this is an effective way of changing behaviour. For example, use the telephone, text messaging, apps or the internet.

Recommendation 8

Ensure interventions meet individual needs

Providers of behaviour change programmes and interventions and trained behaviour change practitioners should:

- Ensure service users are given clear information on the behaviour change interventions and services available and how to use them. If necessary, they should help people to access the services.

- Ensure services are acceptable to, and meet, service users' needs. This includes any needs in relation to a disability or another 'protected characteristic' in relation to equity.

- Recognise the times when people may be more open to change, such as when recovering from a behaviour-related condition (for example, following diagnosis of cardiovascular disease) or when becoming a parent. Also recognise when offering a behaviour change intervention may not be appropriate due to personal circumstances.

Trained behaviour change practitioners (see recommendations 12 and 13) should:

- Before starting an intervention:
    - Assess participants' health in relation to the behaviour and the type of actions needed.
    - For example, they should ensure the level and type of physical activity recommended is appropriate, bearing in mind the person's physical health. (As an example, see Weight management before, during and after pregnancy, NICE public health guidance 27).
    - Ensure the intensity of the intervention matches the person's need for support to change their behaviour.
    - Discuss what the likely impact will be if the participant makes changes to their behaviour (in terms of their health and wellbeing and the health and wellbeing with those they are in contact with).

- Plan at what point before, during and after a behaviour change intervention a review will be undertaken to assess progress towards goals and then tailor the intervention and follow-up support accordingly.

- Tailor interventions to meet participants' needs by assessing and then addressing:
- People's behaviour: if available, use a validated assessment tool appropriate for the specific population or setting. For example, alcohol screening tools used in prisons are different from those used in accident and emergency departments.
- Participants' physical and psychological capability to make change.
- The context in which they live and work (that is, their physical, economic and social environment).
- How motivated they are to change: if many behaviours need to be changed, assess which one – or ones – the person is most motivated to tackle (see Capability, opportunity and motivation).
- Any specific needs with regards to sexual orientation, gender identity, gender, culture, faith or any type of disability.

Recommendation 9

Deliver very brief, brief, extended brief and high intensity behaviour change interventions and programmes

Commissioners and providers of behaviour change services should:

- Encourage health, wellbeing and social care staff (see Who should take action?) in direct contact with the general public to use a very brief intervention to motivate people to change behaviours that may damage their health. The interventions should also be used to inform people about services or interventions that can help them improve their general health and wellbeing.

- Encourage staff who regularly come into contact with people whose health and wellbeing could be at risk to provide them with a brief intervention. (The risk could be due to current behaviours, socio-demographic characteristics or family history.)

- Encourage behaviour change service providers and other health and social care staff dealing with the general public to provide an extended brief intervention to people they regularly see for 30 minutes or more who:

  - are involved in risky behaviours (for example higher risk drinking)

  - have a number of health problems

  - have been assessed as being at increased or higher risk of harm

  - have been successfully making changes to their behaviour but need more support to maintain that change

  - have found it difficult to change or have not benefited from a very brief or brief intervention.

- Encourage behaviour change service providers and practitioners to provide high intensity interventions (typically these last more than 30 minutes and are delivered over a number of sessions) for people they regularly work with who:

  - have been assessed as being at high risk of causing harm to their health and wellbeing (for example, adults with a BMI more than 40 – see Obesity, NICE clinical guideline 43) and/or

- have a serious medical condition that needs specialist advice and monitoring (for example, people with type 2 diabetes or cardiovascular disease) and/or
- have not benefited from lower-intensity interventions (for example, an extended brief intervention).

Recommendation 10

Ensure behaviour change is maintained for at least a year

Providers and practitioners involved with behaviour change programmes and interventions should help people maintain their behaviour change in the long term (more than 1 year) by ensuring they:

- receive feedback and monitoring at regular intervals for a minimum of 1 year after they complete the intervention (the aim is to make sure they can get help if they show any sign of relapse)
- have well-rehearsed action plans (such as if-then plans) that they can easily put into practice if they relapse
- have thought about how they can make changes to their own immediate physical environment to prevent a relapse
- have the social support they need to maintain changes
- are helped to develop routines that support the new behaviour (note that small, manageable changes to daily routine are most likely to be maintained).

Recommendation 11

Commission training for all staff involved in helping to change people's behaviour

Commissioners, local education and training boards, and managers and supervisors (see Who should take action?) should:

- Commission training for relevant staff to meet the service specification for any behaviour change intervention or programme. This should:
  - cover all the various activities, from a very brief intervention offered when the opportunity arises to extended brief interventions
  - include assessment of people's behaviours and needs
  - address equity issues
  - provide the latest available evidence of effectiveness and describe how an intervention works (mechanism of action).
- Ensure training programmes on behaviour change provide:
  - evidence-based content (see recommendation 7)
  - evidence-based training methods
  - trainers with proven skills, knowledge and experience (competencies) in the particular area (see recommendation 12)
  - monitoring using relevant behaviour change competency frameworks or assessment.

Commissioners and local education and training boards should:

- Ensure training programmes consider:
  - where programmes and interventions will be delivered
  - training participants' characteristics (such as background)
  - whether behaviour change is part of participants' main role, integral to their role but not the main focus, or an additional task (see recommendation 9).
- Ensure training includes on going professional development on how to encourage behaviour change. This could include regular refresher training to maintain the quality of delivery of behaviour change interventions.
- Ensure training is evaluated in terms of outcomes (see recommendation 14) and process (for example, via participant feedback).

Recommendation 12

Provide training for behaviour change practitioners

Providers of behaviour change training should:

- Ensure training objectives include the range of knowledge and skills (competences) needed to deliver specific interventions.

- Ensure practitioners are trained to adopt a person-centred approach when assessing people's needs and planning and developing an intervention for them.

- Ensure behaviour change practitioners:

  - understand the factors that may affect behaviour change, including the psychological, social, cultural and economic factors (see recommendation 8)

  - are aware of behaviours that adversely affect people's health and wellbeing, and the benefits of prevention and management can address health inequalities by tailoring interventions to people's specific needs, including their cultural, social and economic needs and other "protected characteristics"

  - are able to assess people's needs and can help select appropriate evidence-based interventions

  - know how an intervention works (mechanism of action)

  - recognise the specific behaviour change techniques used in the intervention they will be delivering

  - understand how to access, and how to direct and refer people to, specialist support services (for example, they should know how people can get help to change their behaviour after hospitalisation, a routine GP appointment or an intervention)

  - understand local policy and demographics.

- Ensure behaviour change practitioners have the skills to:

  - assess people's behaviour using validated assessment tools and measures

  - communicate effectively, for example, by giving people health, wellbeing and other information, by using reflective listening and knowing how to show empathy

- develop rapport and relationships with service users
- develop a person's motivation to change by encouraging and enabling them to manage their own behaviour (see recommendation 7)
- deliver the relevant behaviour change techniques
- help prevent and manage relapses (see recommendation 10).
- Ensure behaviour change practitioners who provide interventions to groups can:
  - elicit group discussions
  - provide group tasks that promote interaction or bonding
  - encourage mutual support within the group.
- Give practitioners the opportunity to learn how to tailor interventions to meet the needs and preferences of different groups and to test this ability (both during and after training).
- Ensure trainers have adequate time and resources to assess participants' motivation, skills, confidence and knowledge when they are delivering interventions to particular groups.

Recommendation 13

Provide training for health and social care practitioners

All those who train or accredit health and social care professionals (see Who should take action?) should:

- Ensure behaviour change knowledge, skills and delivery techniques comprise a formal element of initial training, work placements and on going continuous professional development for all those who deliver health and social care services. (See recommendation 12 for details of training content.)

- Ensure all health and social care professionals can, as a minimum, deliver a very brief intervention. (Training modules can be found online, for example, see the National Centre for Smoking Cessation and Training's very brief advice training module.)

Recommendation 14

Assess behaviour change practitioners and provide feedback

Providers of behaviour change training should:

- Assess the ability of trainees to deliver behaviour change techniques and tailor interventions to meet people's needs.

Employers (this includes workplace managers, supervisors and mentors of trainees) should:

- Ensure behaviour change practitioners who have received training are regularly assessed on their ability to deliver behaviour change interventions. This ranges from a very brief intervention to a high intensity intervention (the latter typically lasts longer than 30 minutes and is delivered over multiple sessions). Assessment should reflect the intervention content. It should also include practitioners' ability to provide participants with behaviour change techniques and to tailor interventions to participants' needs. In addition, it should include service user feedback.

Providers of behaviour change training and employers should:

- Ideally, record behaviour change sessions as part of the assessment. Intervention components, such as behaviour change techniques, should be identified in transcripts. Audio or video recording equipment could be used. If this is not possible then, as a minimum, a reliable observation tool should be used to record the intervention. An example of the latter would be a checklist of key intervention components.

- Obtain the consent of the practitioner and service user for all assessments. They should also ensure the organisation's confidentiality requirements are met.

- Provide behaviour change practitioners with feedback on their performance, both orally and in writing, starting with feedback on good performance. If necessary, negotiate and set jointly agreed goals and an action plan. Provide them with the option of refresher training.

Recommendation 15

Monitor behaviour change interventions

- Commissioners, providers and researchers (see Who should take action?) should ensure all interventions are monitored in terms of:
  - process measures (for example, uptake and reach of the intervention)
  - impact on health inequalities
  - behavioural outcomes in the short, medium and long-term
  - how closely they follow the intervention manual (intervention fidelity) (see recommendation 6).
- If possible, providers should adapt existing electronic systems to collect data on the behaviour of participants. For an example of what could be collected on smoking, see the National Centre for Smoking Cessation and Training stop smoking service client record form.

Recommendation 16

Evaluate behaviour change interventions

- Before introducing a new intervention, commissioners and providers of behaviour change interventions and researchers should be clear about the objectives and how these will be measured and evaluated. (Researchers could include practitioners and others, for more details see Who should take action?) See Medical Research Council guidance on the development, evaluation and implementation of complex interventions to improve health.

- Commissioners and providers should ensure evaluation is carried out by a team of researchers or an organisation that has not been involved in delivering the intervention.

- Researchers should work with commissioners and providers to plan evaluation before the intervention takes place. This may entail getting specialist input (for example, from the NIHR research design service).

- Researchers should use objective, validated measures of outcome and process if they are available. They should ensure the design makes it possible to provide new evidence of effectiveness and, ideally, cost effectiveness – and details on why it is effective (mechanism of action). See principles 7 and 8 in "Behaviour change: the principles for effective interventions" (NICE public health guidance 6).

- Commissioners, providers and researchers should ensure evaluation includes:
  - a description of the evaluation design
  - assessment of intervention fidelity
  - consistent use of valid, reliable measures (using the same tools to assess behaviours) before, during and following an intervention (that is, ensuring baseline and outcome measures match)
  - rigorous qualitative assessments to evaluate how well interventions will work in practice and how acceptable they are to services users and practitioners
  - assessment of processes and outcomes using both objective and self-reported measures
  - establishing and ensuring routine data collection
  - adequate sample sizes
  - assessment of long-term outcomes (more than 1 year).

- Providers of existing interventions should work with researchers to ensure they are rigorously evaluated.

Latest advice on alcohol limits should be accessed (see guidance from the Chief Medical Officer). At publication of this guidance, government advice states that men should not regularly drink more than 3–4 units a day and women should not regularly drink more than 2–3 units a day (see the Change 4 Life website). Regularly drinking 22–50 units per week (men) or 15–35 units per week (women) is described as "increasing-risk drinking". Regularly drinking more than 50 alcohol units per week (men) or more than 35 units per week (women) is described as "higher risk drinking".

Further guidance on behaviour change

Recently, two useful guides to one-to-one behaviour change interventions have been published that are relevant to the dental team[8,9]. In addition the third edition of *Delivering better oral health: an evidence-based toolkit for prevention*[1] includes a section on "Helping patients to change their behaviour". The use of motivational interviewing, as a non-judgmental, non-confrontational and non-adversarial counselling method is now being advocated. This approach attempts to increase the client's awareness of the potential problems caused, consequences experienced, and risks faced as a result of the behaviour in question[10].

Which topics are included in this document?

Over the years, many requests had been received to include additional topics within *The Scientific Basis of Oral Health Education* document. To understand the problems involved in selecting topics for inclusion, it is helpful to consider possible topics under three headings:

- Topics where a substantial body of scientific evidence is available to support a useful health education statement, an example being the use of fluoride toothpaste.

- Topics where guidance for the public in the form of a health education message is required but where scientific evidence is lacking. Provided that there is a consensus of scientific opinion, a statement can be made, though this will be subject to change as new evidence and guidelines are published. An example being how often people should have a dental check-up.

- Topics that require guidance for the public but where there is neither a substantial body of scientific evidence nor a consensus of opinion amongst experts. If experts cannot agree then no statement can or should be given. An example is whether the teeth should be brushed before or after eating.

The nature of scientific evidence

Scientific evidence comes in many forms, but in the context of oral health it breaks down into two main categories:

Laboratory-based studies

These range from purely chemical or biological observations and experiments on the structure of teeth and the mouth, to experiments involving animals or small groups of human volunteers. Examples include the analysis of the changes that occur in teeth when they decay, and studies on the effect on bacteria in the mouth when human volunteers use different types of toothpaste.

Clinical studies

These include observational studies where existing aspects of health are studied in large groups or populations without any form of intervention. Observational studies can include longitudinal ones where a group of subjects are followed over a period of time, cross-sectional studies and case-control studies where a comparison is made with a control group. An important type of clinical study is the interventional experiment. These studies are usually made up of at least two groups, one of which will be a control group who received no intervention and the other groups will follow some form of experimental regime. A good example is the clinical trial of a new toothpaste. In an ideal experiment, subjects will be randomly allocated to a group and the research workers who make the observations will have no knowledge of the group to which any subject has been allocated. This type of experiment is called a randomised controlled trial (RCT) and has often been described as the gold standard for clinical research. Clinical scientists begin with what is called a 'null hypothesis', which means that no difference between the test and control groups is anticipated. The experiment, be it in the test tube or in the form of a RCT aims to blindly "break" or "disprove" that hypothesis.

Good research studies are usually published in peer-reviewed scientific and clinical journals. These accept only those manuscripts which have been reviewed independently and refereed by experts in the field to ensure that the methods used and the conclusion that have been drawn are valid. A very useful overview of research in any particular field is often provided by a systematic review. This is usually written by leading experts who look at all the research that has been done on a particular topic or subject, compare and contrast the results, possibly commenting on the quality of the research and draw appropriate conclusions. Evidence from comprehensive systematic reviews has come to occupy a key position between research and practice. Consequently, they have become very influential as a foundation for preventive practice and policy in dentistry. Finally, there is a method of comparing quantitatively the results from a number of studies that have looked at the same issue, usually in the form of randomised controlled trials. Using a sophisticated statistical analysis, the results from all of the trials are pooled together to arrive at one main result. This type of overall analysis of results is called a meta-analysis. By including a meta-analysis in a systematic review it is possible to provide valuable insights concerning the effectiveness of health care interventions.

One very important point must be made about the result of any scientific research. When the conclusion of a study is that 'there is no evidence to form a conclusion', it does not mean that the negative situation has been firmly established. It simply means that the study has not provided evidence for or against the relationship being studied. This is a point that is frequently misunderstood by those without a scientific background, who will reasonably assume that when a scientist says that there is no evidence for this or that, it means that it is not true. All the scientist is saying is that the experiment does not give sufficient evidence to draw a firm conclusion. It is possible that next week or next year evidence will appear that does establish the case.

Health education and evidence-based dentistry

From the early 1970s there has been a growing interest in placing all aspects of clinical practice on an evidence-supported basis. One of the pioneers of this movement was Professor Archie Cochrane, who gave his name to an international collaborative network of groups with the aim of developing evidence-based decision-making for clinical interventions. The Cochrane Collaboration produces a series of systematic reviews of scientific evidence on a range of topics in all areas of health care and some of these are used to support statements made in this document. A further extension of this movement is the appearance of a number of organisations and networks whose aim is to standardise and integrate the methods used for the development of guidelines for clinical practice. In the United Kingdom one of the most useful is that developed by the Scottish Inter-collegiate Guidelines

Network (www.sdcep.org.uk). One result of this work has been to establish a framework that enables those involved in producing clinical guidelines to formulate them on a common basis.

The concept of putting clinical practice on to an evidence basis has run in parallel with work to ensure that health education messages given to the public are based on sound scientific evidence. Nevertheless, an important difference between these two areas is that while the evidence for clinical interventions ideally comes from high quality clinical studies such as randomised controlled trials (RCT), the evidence to support dental health education messages often comes from other types of studies. A system for indicating levels of evidence about the effectiveness of health care interventions has been developed by the Centre for Evidence-based Medicine levels (CEM) and adopted by various evidence-based guidelines organisations worldwide and this scheme is undergoing constant refinement (www.cebm.net). In this book, a simple scheme is introduced to give an indication of the strength of evidence supporting key statements for dental health education and is referred to as Evidence Bases. The equivalent nearest the Centre for Evidence-based Medicine levels (CEM) are given in brackets.

- Evidence Base A: Statements supported by randomised controlled trials, meta-analyses or systematic reviews (CEM levels 1 and 2).
- Evidence Base B: Statements supported by the majority of other relevant studies. (CEM level 3 and 4).
- Evidence Base C: Statements that cannot be supported by a substantial body of research evidence, but where there is a consensus of scientific and professional opinion to support the statement. There may nevertheless be dissenting views, as the issue may be the subject of continuing debate and on going research studies. (CEM level 5).

Where appropriate these grades are marked as Evidence Bases A, B and C, respectively and each would represent the highest grade of evidence that currently exists for a given statement.

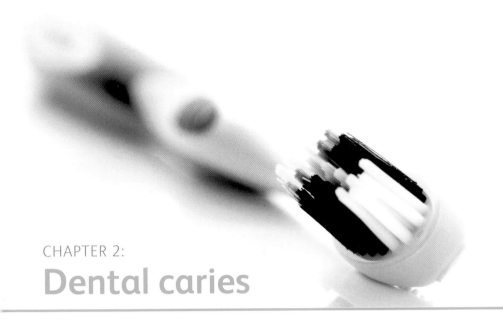

CHAPTER 2

Dental caries

Key points

- Caries occurs in all populations and age groups.
  Evidence Base A

- Caries is caused by the action of sugars on the bacterial plaque covering the teeth.
  Evidence Base A

- The risk of developing caries can be reduced by avoiding sugars between meals and at bedtime.
  Evidence Base B

- Water fluoridation is safe and effective and is the only means of caries prevention that does not require personal compliance, but may be associated with an increase in mild enamel fluorosis.
  Evidence Base A

- The risk of developing caries can be reduced by brushing with a fluoride toothpaste twice daily, but this requires compliance.
  Evidence Base A

- A pea-sized amount of fluoride toothpaste should be used by young children (a small smear for babies) and brushing should be supervised.
  Evidence Base B

- Supervised brushing of children's teeth with a fluoride toothpaste leads to enhanced caries reduction.
  Evidence Base A

- Fluoride varnish applied twice yearly is effective in helping to prevent caries.
  Evidence Base A

- Never leave infants with sugars-sweetened drinks in feeding bottles or cups, especially at bedtime.
  Evidence Base B

Who gets caries?

This condition is often said to be one of the most common diseases affecting mankind. This was true for much of the Western developed world during the last century, but not for Asia and Africa. Within Europe and North America, the level of caries in children appeared to reach a peak in the 1960s and decreased in prevalence during the following 30 years. However, during the past decade, the situation has reversed and numerous scientific reports signal an alarming increase in the global prevalence of dental caries in children and adults, both in primary and permanent teeth, as well as coronal and root surfaces[11].

While it remains a major health problem for people of all ages, its peak activity occurs during childhood. In China, Mexico and the Philippines, prevalence of more than 90% in young children has been reported. In the UK national surveys were undertaken at regular intervals by the NHS in partnership with the British Association for the Study of Community Dentistry. Since 2012 oral health surveys in England have been administered by Public Health England. The 2011/12 survey showed that 27.9% of five-year-old children in England examined with parental consent had experienced dental caries, on average affecting 3.4 of their teeth[12]. The average number of affected teeth in the whole sample (including the 72.1% who were free of dental caries) was 0.9. The results from the 2011/12 Welsh survey showed that 41% of five-year-olds had dental caries on average affecting 3.8 teeth[13]. The results from the 2011/12 Scottish survey showed 33% of five-year-olds had decay experience[14]. An interesting comparison comes from the 2002 North – South survey of children's dental health in Ireland. In the Republic of Ireland where 70% of the population is supplied with artificially fluoridated water, 5-year olds in the fluoridated areas had on average one decayed tooth. In non-fluoridated Northern Ireland 5-years olds had 1.8 decayed teeth. For 15 year olds the figures were 2.1 and 3.6 respectively[15].

There are wide variations in caries prevalence, often within small geographical areas and this is related to two social factors. Firstly, like many other diseases, it has become apparent that a high level of dental caries is essentially a disease associated with social deprivation. In the UK, a low prevalence of dental caries can now be seen in the more affluent areas, especially in southern England. However, levels remain high in children in many inner city socially deprived areas of Wales, Scotland and Northern Ireland, and northern parts of England. The second factor is ethnicity and is a complex one, possibly related to different dietary and toothbrushing practices within different cultures. Some children of Asian ethnic background, including children of non-English speaking mothers, have the highest caries rates for primary teeth. One UK study of five-year olds found that Asian children had 60% more decayed teeth than white children living in the same towns[16]. However, this difference is not apparent in the permanent teeth of older children.

How caries affects teeth

Dental caries affects the tooth itself. The consequences of caries are familiar to most people (Fig 2.1). The process begins at the tooth surface but is often hidden from sight in the fissures (grooves) or between the teeth. Where it is visible the initial appearance may be as a chalky white patch or ring around the neck of the tooth or as a shadow or staining on the biting surface (Fig. 2.2).

The chalky appearance is due to the enamel surface having lost some of the calcium and phosphate mineral crystals of which it is largely composed. This process is called demineralisation. The destructive process can then spread

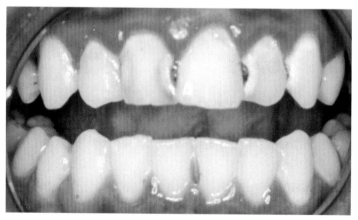

Fig.2.1   Dental caries.

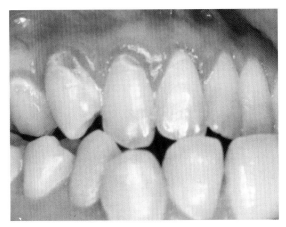

Fig. 2.2   Caries at the necks of teeth, from 'white spot' stage to cavitation.

into the dentine (the softer, sensitive part of the tooth beneath the enamel). The weakened enamel then collapses to form a cavity and the tooth is progressively destroyed. Dental caries causes progressive destruction of the crowns of the teeth often accompanied by severe pain and infection. The roots of teeth can also be attacked should they become exposed by gum recession and this is more common in older adults.

Cause

The basic process that causes caries is sometimes called an 'acid attack'. Caries begins within the plaque on the tooth surface following the consumption of sugars in drinks and foods.

- When sugars enter the mouth they are rapidly absorbed by the bacteria in the plaque layer on the surfaces of the teeth.
- Inside the bacterial cells the sugars are converted by metabolic processes into organic acids as a waste product and excreted into the plaque fluid.
- The acids accumulate in the plaque layer and cause demineralisation of the enamel surface.

SUGARS → PLAQUE → ACID → DEMINERALISATION

This 'acid attack' is more accurately described as a 'demineralisation episode' caused by the action of plaque bacteria on sugars entering the mouth. Sucrose and glucose are the most important dietary sugars as they are added to many food products and beverages during manufacture. As table sugar, sucrose is often added during cooking or immediately before consumption. These simple sugars can enter the plaque bacteria and be metabolised within minutes of being consumed. Since plaque covers most tooth surfaces and reforms quickly after brushing, acid forms within the plaque in contact with the teeth. Most people will consume some sugars as part of the everyday diet, but not everyone develops caries. To explain why this is so we must look in more detail at the factors that determine the risk from dental caries. The pattern and severity of attack are determined by two groups of factors – those in the environment of the tooth, which influence the severity of the attack and those factors that influence the tooth's resistance to attack.

The tooth's environment

The important factors within the mouth that interact to influence the severity of attack are plaque, dietary sugars, saliva and fluoride. Sugars from the diet pass into the plaque within seconds of consumption. Many plaque bacteria use sugars as their source of energy and rapidly produce acid as a by-product. As acid is generated, it accumulates in the plaque layer and acidity in the plaque increases. Acidity is measured on the pH scale, and the lower the figure, the greater the degree of acidity. Figure 2.3 shows the effect of a sugar intake on plaque pH. The fall in plaque pH when sugars enter the mouth and the subsequent recovery as shown in the diagram is called the 'Stephan curve'. This demineralisation-remineralisation episode is sometimes referred to as an 'acid attack'. Within minutes of a sugar intake, sufficient acid may be generated within the absorbent plaque layer to cause a small outflow of calcium and phosphate from the enamel resulting in a tiny degree of demineralisation. After a period of time (usually about 20 minutes, but possibly up to two hours), the acid will have dissipated and the lost mineral may be slowly replaced from the saliva. This process is called remineralisation. However, if sugars are consumed frequently during the day, especially without the presence of other food or liquids that might dilute or help neutralise the acid, then the amount of demineralisation may exceed remineralisation.

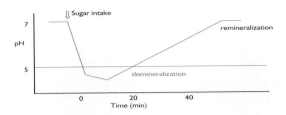

Fig. 2.3   The effect of sugar intake on plaque pH.

This situation is illustrated in Figure 2.4a where a frequent intake of sugars during the day leads to an unfavorable proportion of total demineralization to remineralisation periods, while an infrequent sugars intake results in a more favorable proportion as seen in Figure 2.4b. If this imbalance persists over a period of time, then the gradual loss of mineral from the enamel may lead to its eventual breakdown and the formation of a cavity.

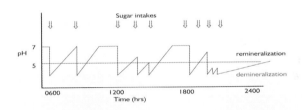

Fig. 2.4a   Frequency of sugars intake.

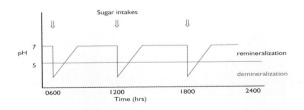

Fig. 2.4b   Benefits of infrequent sugars intake.

The type of bacteria that predominate within the plaque is influenced by the diet. Frequent consumption of sugars has been shown to encourage the multiplication of bacteria that use sugars and can efficiently convert them to acid and it also increases the thickness of the plaque layer. The most commonly implicated plaque organism is Streptococcus mutans, however there are many other types that metabolise sugars to form acid. The proportion of these caries-causing bacteria falls when the amount and frequency of dietary sugars are reduced.

However, the mouth has its own defense mechanisms. While these are not fully understood, saliva is clearly the most important as it bathes the plaque on the tooth surface and helps to neutralise the acids and wash away sugars.

This effect is enhanced if salivary flow after sugary snacks is stimulated for example by vegetables, cheese or sugar-free chewing gum. In addition, at the very earliest stages of the decay process, the tooth surface may "heal" or "remineralise" by deposition from saliva of calcium and phosphate, together with fluoride, which accelerates the healing process. The early caries process may be seen as a contest fought at the tooth surface between the acids (resulting from the intake of sugars) causing demineralisation of the tooth surface and a number of factors including fluoride and saliva promoting the remineralisation of the tooth surface.

It is now well established that plaque matures as it is left to grow within the mouth. Moments after the teeth are brushed a layer of protein, called the pellicle, forms. The tooth becomes covered in protein and within minutes plaque bacteria can begin to colonise the pellicle. With time, the plaque becomes thicker and will contain a more diverse colony of many bacteria. Particularly if the diet is rich in sugars, the plaque grows and reaches its most mature at about seven days. Plaque of this age will break down the sugars extremely quickly, again putting the mineral component of the tooth in danger of becoming demineralised. This mature plaque layer is often referred to as a "biofilm" since it can be made of several hundred types of bacteria that will change in type from the tooth surface to the outer surface of the plaque.

Diet

Sugars in our diet

While there are several dietary sugars that have been linked to caries, sucrose is the most important. Food industry statistics estimate that almost half of the sucrose consumed by the public is sold as packaged sugar and about half is used by food, drink and confectionery manufacturers. The major industrial use of sucrose is the production of confectionery, which accounts for about a quarter of the total used in manufacturing, while the soft drinks industry uses about one fifth.

Nearly three-quarters of all sugars in the UK diet are added to foods during manufacture, cooking or before consumption. Confectionery, soft drinks, cakes, biscuits and table sugar (in tea and coffee, for example) are often consumed between meals and their frequent consumption is strongly linked to dental caries. The other sugars in the diet are naturally present in foods such as whole fruit, vegetables and milk. When sugars are consumed as part of these foods they are considered to be relatively unimportant as a cause of decay.

Dietary advice

Dietary advice should be aimed at changing the pattern of consumption of sugars with the aim of reducing the frequency and amount of consumption. Food and drinks containing added sugars should be identified and restricted, especially between meals. While fresh fruit and vegetables naturally contain sugars, their consumption as part of a normal diet is not linked to caries and they have an important place in our diet. People should be encouraged to eat snacks that are sugar-free (e.g. carrots, peppers, breadsticks, savoury sandwiches and cheese). Fresh fruit is a really important part of the diet, however fruit juice and dried fruit can adversely affect teeth because of their high concentration of sugars and acid and are not recommended for consumption between meals. Concentrated fruit juices and cordials should be well diluted with water. Plain water and milk are the safest drinks as far as the teeth are concerned.

Parents and careers of infants should be warned of the dangers of putting fruit juice or sugars-sweetened drinks into feeding bottles, valve-type or reservoir feeders for the child to hold, especially in bed. Such practices result in almost continuous bathing of the enamel with sugars and can lead to rapid tooth destruction. From six months of age, infants should be introduced to drinking from a cup. Free-flowing lidded feeding cups can help avoid spills in the early stages, before infants move on to an open beaker or cup. Feeding bottles should be given up completely after the age of 12 months.

People should also be encouraged to study the nutritional labels of food and drinks, and avoid frequently consuming those with high levels of sugars such as those containing more than 10g per 100g. Foods and drinks may contain added sugars other than sucrose. The ingredient of greatest amount is always listed first and the words used to describe sugars include glucose, maltose, fructose, hydrolysed starch, invert sugar, corn syrup and honey (when listed as an added sugar). They are as likely as sucrose to cause caries and should not be used in infant drinks and foods unless they are consumed only at mealtimes. If one of these is near the top of the list of ingredients the food or drink is likely to be high in sugars. Colour-coded nutritional information on many products tells the consumer at a glance if the food has high, medium or low amounts of fat, saturated fat, sugars and salt.

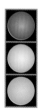

red means high

amber means medium

green means low

In short, the more green lights, the healthier the choice.

The use of sugars in medicines should also be strongly discouraged and sugar-free liquid medicines should be chosen by prescribers and when buying non-prescription medicines, whenever possible. If children have a long-term medical condition, parents and careers should request clinicians to prescribe sugar-free liquid medicines or preferably, tablets instead of liquids.

Preferable snacks and drinks for between-meal consumption

For between-meal snacks and drinks, raw vegetables such as carrots, fresh fruit, brown or wholemeal bread, low-fat unsweetened yoghurt, lower-fat cheese, skimmed or semi- skimmed milk and water can be recommended. Whole cow's milk should only be used as a main milk drink after the age of one year. Children between one and two years of age need whole milk. Between the ages of two and five years, provided they are eating a good varied diet, semi-skimmed milk can be introduced. Skimmed milk should not be given before the age of five. Milk and water are the only safe drinks for the teeth. Fruit juices contain sugars and acids, so it's best to have these only at mealtimes. Fruit juice should be diluted with 10 parts water to 1 of juice. Babies under 6 months should not be given fruit juices or cordials. More information on diet and caries can be found in Chapter 3.

The tooth's resistance

Largely because of their shape or position in the mouth some teeth are more resistant to attack than others. For example, in young people lower front teeth rarely decay because they don't have any grooves or fissures in which plaque can stagnate and they are bathed by saliva, which is beneficial. In contrast, the first permanent molar teeth have the highest decay rate because the deep fissures on the biting surfaces are difficult to clean. The one factor that has been shown beyond doubt to reduce the rate of dental caries is fluoride and this is described below. In the UK, neither malnutrition in the mother during pregnancy nor in the child after birth is likely to have any appreciable effect on the susceptibility of the teeth to caries. Calcium cannot be removed from the mother's teeth by the foetus during pregnancy or during lactation.

Prevention

There are two principal ways for individuals to reduce the risk of caries. The first is to reduce the severity of attack by decreasing the frequency and amount of consumption of sugars as described above and in Chapter 3. The second is by using fluoride, easily and effectively done by brushing twice-daily with a fluoride-containing toothpaste. These methods should be used together in order to improve and maintain oral health.

Fluoride

Fluoride toothpaste

Fluoride toothpaste, which came into general use in the USA in the 1950s and in Europe and the UK in the early 1970s, is now recognised as a development of the greatest importance to dental health. It is thought to be the most cost-effective topical fluoride agent for personal use and is likely to be the main reason for the decline in caries prevalence in Europe and most developed countries during the last 30 years. The daily use of a fluoride toothpaste containing at least 1,000 parts per million (ppm) fluoride is a highly effective method of delivering fluoride to the tooth surface and to some extent its use has removed the need for professionally applied fluoride agents, except in special circumstances. In the UK fluoride toothpastes are currently available in three concentration ranges: standard pastes containing about 1,000–1,500 ppm and high concentration pastes containing over 2,000 ppm. Low fluoride formulations containing 500 - 600 ppm were introduced to meet the concern that young children might ingest excessive fluoride. Research has shown that the effectiveness of fluoride toothpastes increases with the fluoride concentration and there is no clear evidence that pastes containing less than 1,000 ppm are effective[17], however the use of higher concentration fluoride toothpastes by children have been associated with an increase in dental fluorosis. The Department of Health in England now advises that children under 3 years of age should use a toothpaste containing at least 1,000 ppm, but that only a thin smear of paste (equivalent to half a pea-size) be applied on the brush[1]. For maximum benefit children aged 3 years and older and adults should use a toothpaste containing 1,350 – 1,500 ppm, but these standard pastes should not be used by children who might eat or swallow the paste. For children from 3 to 6 years of age care should be taken to apply only a pea-sized amount and parents must ensure that children do not eat or lick fluoride toothpaste from the tube. Parents should supervise and finish off the brushing to ensure that an appropriate amount of toothpaste is applied and that the child does not ingest the toothpaste. The labeling of toothpastes remains unsatisfactory as the total fluoride content is not clearly marked in a simple form for the public to recognise.

While brands with similar fluoride concentrations may be equally effective, other components of the formulation may influence overall benefit. A number of leading brands have been independently evaluated in published long-term clinical trials in order to ensure efficacy. There is evidence that rinsing with water immediately after brushing with fluoride toothpaste reduces the benefit both in relation to the development of new cavities and the prevention of recurrent caries around fillings. It is preferable simply to spit out the excess paste. When fluoride drops or tablets are used (see below) they should be given at a different time of day to brushing and rinsing with a fluoride mouthrinse if used.

Water fluoridation

Fluorides are compounds of the chemical element fluorine. They are widely found in nature, in some foods such as fish (bones), in some plants such as tea, in beer and in some natural water supplies. The link between the presence of fluoride in public water supplies, enamel mottling (fluorosis) and reduced caries experience was first noticed early last century and has been demonstrated by over 130 surveys in more than 20 countries including the UK. These surveys showed that fluoride in the water at a concentration of about one part per million (1 ppm) reduces caries levels by up to half compared to similar non-fluoride areas. In 1945, Grand Rapids in the USA became the first community to have its water supply artificially adjusted to contain 1 ppm fluoride. Since then many cities around the world have followed, the largest schemes in the UK being in Birmingham, including parts of the West Midlands, and Newcastle upon Tyne. Worldwide, about 370 million people are supplied with artificially fluoridated water – an increase of 20 million people over the past ten years and 27 countries operate fluoridation schemes. In addition, an estimated 50 million people drink water whose naturally occurring fluoride is at the optimum concentration. Over 90% of the population of Australia and 70% of the populations of the USA, the Republic of Ireland, Israel and several other countries have water fluoridation.

The safety of water fluoridation is well documented. Numerous studies in both natural and artificially fluoridated areas have failed to show any adverse effect on general health at the level of 1 ppm, although fluoridation may be associated with an increase in dental fluorosis. One of the most authoritative reports is that of the Royal College of Physicians of England (1976). Fluoride's effectiveness and safety were upheld in the Court of Session judgment in Edinburgh in 1983. In 2011 a report by the EU Commission's Scientific Committee on Health and Environmental Risks (SCHER) concluded on the basis of the latest available evidence that "exposure of environmental organisms to the levels of fluoride used for fluoridation of drinking water is not expected to lead to unacceptable risks to the environment".

At an international level, water fluoridation is supported by the World Health Organisation (WHO), the Fédération Dentaire Internationale (FDI) and the International Association for Dental Research (IADR) as a safe and effective means of reducing dental caries. The US Centers for Disease Control and Prevention has recognised fluoridation as one of 10 great public health achievements of the 20th Century and the American Dental Association and the US Surgeon-General have reaffirmed their support for water fluoridation (2013). Within the UK, water fluoridation has been embodied in guidance documents from the UK Department of Health, including An Oral Health Strategy for England (1994) and Modernising NHS Dentistry – Implementing the NHS Plan (2000), It was supported by the All Party Parliamentary Primary Care & Public Health Group (2003) and in England and Wales it is embodied in the Water Act 2004. UK professional bodies supporting water fluoridation include the Royal Society of Public Health, the Royal College of Physicians, the British Medical Association, the British Dental Association and the Medical Research Council. A systematic review of water fluoridation by the NHS Centre for Reviews and Dissemination at the University of York (2000) provides a comprehensive review of the knowledge base in this area. It concluded that water fluoridation reduces dental caries incidence by an average of 15%, and that caries prevalence increases following withdrawal of water fluoridation. While water fluoridation was found to reduce inequalities between social groups, by reducing the differences in caries severity among five and 12 year-old children, there was evidence for a slight increase in dental fluorosis levels. Finally, the review found no clear associations between water fluoridation and systemic morbidity[18].

Analysis of the reduction in treatment need after fluoridation has shown savings in manpower and resources. A large fall in the numbers of extractions and general anaesthetics administered to children has been reported by Public Health England in their 2014 health monitoring report (see Further Reading). Furthermore, there is evidence from Scotland that the discontinuation of water fluoridation can result in a return to higher caries levels, despite the benefit of fluoride toothpaste. A 25% increase in caries prevalence was recorded five years after parts of Scotland were de-fluoridated. However, in some countries no change in caries levels has been seen after de-fluoridation. This might be due to changes in diet or the increased use of fluoride toothpaste.

While in some areas falling caries prevalence has reduced the absolute benefit to be gained from water fluoridation, in communities where prevalence remains high, often because of social and economic factors, there are significant potential benefits[19]. Because of these changes, the consensus of expert opinion is that water fluoridation should be targeted at areas with higher caries levels. It must be emphasised that water fluoridation is the only means of caries prevention that does not require personal compliance.

Other fluoride agents

Where additional protection is indicated for erupted teeth, other fluoride containing agents are effective[20]. These include toothpaste containing higher fluoride concentrations, fluoride mouthrinses containing 250 ppm for daily home use and fluoride varnishes containing typically 22,600 ppm which need to be applied by dentists, therapists, hygienists or trained dental nurses every 6 months. Fluoride varnish professionally applied is of proven effectiveness[21] and the Department of Health in England recommends that all children over the age of three have a fluoride varnish application every 6 months[17]. Fluoride mouthrinses are readily available in most countries and have proved effective and convenient for home use[22]. They should be used at a different time of day to toothbrushing and not just before food or drink to maximise benefit, however they are not advised for children under 6 years of age. Like standard toothpaste they provide fluoride to saliva and plaque on tooth surfaces and invoke the first two, and most important, fluoride mechanisms described below. These agents are of greatest value for children at risk to caries and adults suffering from a dry mouth, medically compromised individuals and those undergoing orthodontic treatment.

Fluoride tablets and drops

These were originally introduced to mimic the effect of water fluoridation. A systematic review found that the use of fluoride supplements was associated with a 24% caries reduction in permanent teeth but the effect on primary teeth was unclear. When the fluoride supplements were compared with the use of topically-applied fluorides such as toothpastes, varnishes, and mouthrinses there was no differential effect, on permanent or deciduous teeth. For maximum effectiveness, daily administration from infancy until adolescence was required, although compliance with this regime was recognised as a frequent problem. Fluoride drops and tablets are available on prescription from dentists and doctors in the UK and may be purchased from pharmacists without a prescription. While initially seen as a potential public health measure, the introduction of fluoride toothpaste in the early 1970s has proved to be far more effective. Some experts now doubt the extent of any additional benefit that their use may provide beyond that achieved by effective twice-daily toothbrushing with a fluoride toothpaste[23]. Today, their use should be confined to those at very high risk of caries or to those for whom dental treatment may be complicated by their general or physical condition. These groups include children with heart disease or cardiac defects as well as children prone to infection because of systemic disorders. Children with mental or physical disabilities may be more at risk of dental disease because of oral hygiene and dietary problems and may find dental treatment, when needed, difficult or frightening. All of these children could benefit from fluoride supplements. The need for their use should be determined with dental advice and reviewed at intervals. Parents and careers should be advised of the benefits, and risks, and especially of the long-term commitment, to the use of this measure, and of the importance of safe storage away from the reach of children. A stop-start pattern of use is unlikely to provide significant benefit. The main problem with the use of fluoride dietary supplements is compliance with the required daily regime over the whole period of tooth formation. Some experts believe that compliance is likely to be higher in motivated families where the children may have a low risk of developing caries, while conversely, compliance may be poor in areas of social deprivation where the caries risk and the need for preventive measures is greater.

Because of compliance problems, some clinicians prefer to rely on professionally applied topical fluoride agents such as fluoride varnishes or gels where additional measures are required. Fluoride drops or tablets should not be given in areas that have the optimum level of fluoride in the water supply and parents should therefore seek professional advice before use. Fluoride supplements should be given daily, but the dose must not be increased if days are missed.

It is generally advised that for maximum benefit supplement use should be continued until the appearance of the second molar teeth, usually at about 11 to 12 years of age. However, this advice is based on the pre-eruptive effect of the ingested fluoride. Some experts believe that by allowing the tablets to dissolve slowly in the mouth a more beneficial topical post-eruptive effect may be achieved, both for older children and adults who may be at risk of dental caries.

Fluoridated milk

The use of fluoridated milk for dental caries prevention was first proposed in the 1950s and school-based fluoridated milk programmes are now operating in 4 countries ranging from Russia to Chile where 220,000 children benefit[24]. In the UK over 30,000 children in over 500 schools drink fluoridated milk at school. This is part of a programme that began in 1993 and was established under the direction of the School of Dental Sciences, University of Liverpool. An additional potential benefit is that fluoridated milk may help displace sweetened soft drinks from the refrigerated vending machines found in many schools. UK studies suggest that at the level 0.5mg F per 189 ml of milk there is limited effectiveness and most effect is seen in the permanent dentition, and a systematic review concluded that due to the general lack of randomised evidence more research of good methodological quality is needed[25]. The organisation and maintenance of school-based programmes can pose problems where there is high absenteeism in infant and primary schools, or difficulty with the reliability of the milk distribution process.

Enamel fluorosis

This condition presents as opaque, white or brown areas, lines or flecks in the enamel surface that are most noticeable when they occur on front teeth. While these opacities can be due to a number of causes, one is the ingestion of excessive fluoride during the period of enamel formation. For incisor teeth the period of greatest risk is between 15 and 30 months of age. The more severe, cosmetically unacceptable forms are uncommon in the UK, but may result from the use of fluoride dietary supplements in optimally fluoridated areas or from the eating of fluoride toothpaste in early childhood. The use of fluoride toothpaste in areas with optimally fluoridated water supplies has been shown by surveys using sensitive photographic recording to result in only a small increase in the mildest forms, which mostly pass unnoticed. No increase in moderate or severe forms has yet been detected, and simple techniques are available to improve the appearance of affected teeth. Nevertheless, this is an area of concern to both the public and the dental professions and care should be taken to ensure that young children do not ingest excessive amounts of fluoride toothpaste, especially in fluoridated areas or when fluoride supplements are used[26]. While manufacturers rightly endeavour to make the taste of children's toothpaste attractive, there is concern that the use of food flavouring such as strawberry may encourage excessive consumption.

To reduce the risk of fluorosis, parents should supervise toothbrushing of children under seven years of age and should place an amount of toothpaste no greater than the size of a pea on the brush (or a small smear for babies). Brushing should be done normally no more than twice each day and the child should be encouraged to spit out afterwards, rather than rinse with water. Supervision will continue to be beneficial beyond this age. When fluoride drops or tablets are used, they should be given at a different time of day to brushing.

How does fluoride work?

Teeth and bone are composed largely of a crystalline mineral compound of calcium and phosphate called hydroxyapatite. Research over the past 60 years has shown that fluoride produces its effect in a number of different ways which combine to slow and help prevent the caries process and also to reverse caries in its early stages. These are given below in the order of effectiveness.

- *Enhanced remineralisation* – Very low levels of fluoride in the plaque and saliva are able to alter the chemical balance between demineralisation of the enamel and remineralisation. The effect favours the remineralisation process, allowing the early carious attack on enamel to be reversed and new mineral crystals, with better structure and greater acid resistance, to be deposited. This is the mechanism by which fluoride toothpaste is thought to work and appears to be the most important.
- *Reduced acid production* – Fluoride is concentrated in the plaque layer on the surfaces of the teeth and reduces the conversion of dietary sugars into acid by plaque bacteria. Fluoride toothpaste also invokes this mechanism.
- *Fluoride substitution* – Fluoride entering the developing teeth from the diet via the blood stream is incorporated into the new mineral crystals. The partly fluoridated hydroxyapatite that is formed is theoretically more resistant to acid attack than that formed without fluoride.
- *Reduced pit and fissure depth* – The parts of the teeth most susceptible to caries are the natural pits and grooves, or fissures on the biting surfaces of back teeth. Fluoride entering the developing teeth at an early stage appears to result in reduced pit and fissure depth.

The use of fluoride toothpaste, which delivers its effect at the tooth surface, has reduced the significance of the last two mechanisms, which are now thought to play a minor role.

Plaque control

Dental caries cannot develop without the presence of plaque, which is needed to convert dietary sugars into acid. Some research studies have shown that highly efficient toothbrushing techniques with professional guidance can reduce dental caries. However research has shown that normal "real world" toothbrushing alone does not appear to be as effective. Some plaque is left in fissures and other stagnation sites where caries occurs and plaque reforms rapidly on cleaned tooth surfaces. The use of a fluoride toothpaste is firmly established as the most effective personal means for caries prevention as brushing with a fluoride toothpaste delivers fluoride to the teeth and is the main role of toothbrushing for caries prevention. Nevertheless, the value of effective toothbrushing as the essential means for the prevention of periodontal disease is well established (see Chapter 4). Eating crisp or crunchy foods such as apples or raw carrots will not remove plaque effectively. However they are suitable snack foods and are an important part of a healthy diet. More information on plaque control can be found in Chapter 5.

Fissure sealants

A further way of helping to prevent dental caries is for a plastic film to be professionally applied to the pits and fissures of teeth as soon as possible after the teeth erupt into the mouth. For the permanent molar teeth this is from the age of six years with the eruption of the first permanent molar. The sealant prevents access of plaque and plaque acids to the enamel surface. Clinical trials have shown that sealants can be well retained and prevent caries. However, they are only effective on the biting surfaces of teeth. They are more cost effective in children at higher risk of caries and should be considered when there is a risk to general health from dental caries or dental treatment[27]. In all cases fissure sealants should be seen as one part of a comprehensive preventive plan.

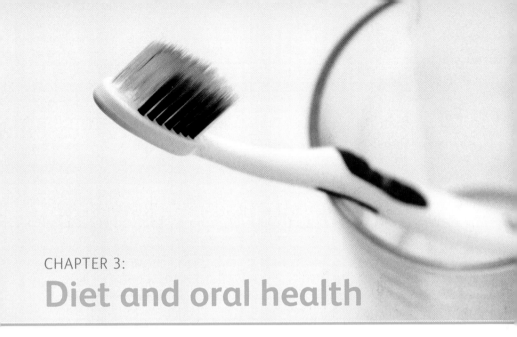

CHAPTER 3:
Diet and oral health

Key points

- The frequency and amount of consumption of sugars in drinks and foods are the most important risk factors for dental caries.
Evidence Base A

- Sugars-sweetened snacks and drinks should be avoided between meals and especially at bedtime.
Evidence Base B

- Naturally occurring sugars, when consumed in fresh whole fruit, vegetables, milk and milk products and cereal grains are not a risk factor for dental caries and these items are an essential part of a healthy balanced diet.
Evidence Base B

Sugars and dental caries

The evidence for a link between sugars and caries comes from a variety of sources. Epidemiological studies have demonstrated a clear correlation between caries experience and mean sugars consumption levels in different countries. The best evidence comes from cohort studies that look at changes in caries over time in relation to sugars intake. When communities have shown changes in sugars consumption, such as during World War II (1939–1945) when consumption fell, a corresponding fall in caries prevalence has been observed. Similarly, groups having low or restricted sugars consumption and those with high consumption of sugars, show corresponding lower or higher levels of caries experience respectively. In children using sugars-sweetened medicines over long periods higher dental caries levels have been found compared to a control group. Human non-randomised clinical studies have demonstrated that when sugars consumption is increased under controlled conditions the caries increment follows and it falls when consumption is reduced. Laboratory studies have demonstrated, by the use of miniature pH electrodes inserted into the plaque on teeth, an immediate fall in pH on the application of a neutral sugar solution, with the acidity persisting for 20 minutes to two hours.

Sugars in food and drinks

The sugars most responsible for dental caries have been classified by the UK Committee on Medical Aspects of Food Policy (COMA, now the Scientific Advisory Committee on Nutrition) as non-milk extrinsic sugars (NMES)[28] as illustrated in Figure 3.1. NMES are those that are added to food and drinks during processing, manufacture or preparation. NMES also include sugars naturally present in fresh fruit juices and fruit concentrates, honey and syrups. The reason that NMES are implicated is that they are simple sugars that can rapidly enter the plaque bacteria and be converted to acid and are often frequently consumed in amounts far in excess of nutritional needs. Sugars naturally present in fruit and vegetables – and eaten as such as part of a normal healthy diet – are not considered to be cariogenic. This is because they are contained within the cell structure of the plant and during mastication may not be fully released into the mouth. Sugars in milk, while extrinsic are not liked to caries risk, although there is some evidence that a pattern of prolonged and extended breastfeeding or leaving an infant with a bottle of milk formula or cow's milk for long periods may pose a risk, especially when the child is asleep. If a child is left with a bottle or comforter (soother) it should only contain water.

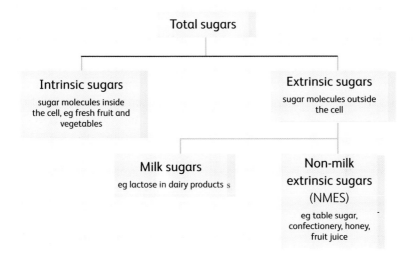

Fig. 3.1   Classification of sugars (COMA, 1989).

Most adults and children in the UK consume too much sugar. The UK National Diet and Nutrition Survey found that mean non-milk extrinsic sugars intakes exceeded the Dietary Reference Value (DRV) (no more than 11% food energy) for children aged four to 18 years and adults aged 19 to 64 years [29]. Soft drinks were the largest contributor to NMES intake for children aged four to 18 years. As the frequency and amount of NMES consumption are strongly linked a reduction in either or preferably both can make a major contribution to the improvement of oral health as well as helping to maintain a healthy diet. Adults and children should not have food and drinks with added sugar more than four times a day and should be encouraged to drink water and low fat milk rather than soft drinks to help reduce sugar intakes.

Fruit and vegetables are an essential part of a healthy diet however all fruit juices have a high concentration of NMES. While these are presently included within the fruit and vegetables recommended by the '5 a day' programme, sponsored by the Department of Health in England, from a dental perspective their frequent consumption especially between meals could increase the risk of dental caries. It should be noted that fresh fruit juices, irrespective of how much is consumed, may each only constitute one of the five daily portions and this point should be stressed when giving dietary advice. Lactose, the sugar in milk, is classed as an NMES if added to other foods or drinks but is less cariogenic than other dietary sugars. When naturally present in milk, it appears to be virtually non-cariogenic.

The common non-milk extrinsic dietary sugars are sucrose (refined from beet and cane), glucose, maltose (extracted from many foods) and fructose (extracted from fruit). Fructose is also a NMES when naturally present in natural unsweetened fruit juice, honey and syrups and when used as an additive to foods and drinks. Significant amounts of glucose and fructose are now made industrially from starch. While sucrose is highly cariogenic, animal studies have shown that both glucose and fructose will readily produce caries and combinations of these sugars appear to be as cariogenic as sucrose alone.

Furthermore, there does not appear to be a safe level for sugars concentration in food and drinks, as this is linked in a complex manner with physical consistency. Indeed, in solution, sucrose concentrations below the taste threshold can generate acid in plaque.

Dietary starch, which is a complex carbohydrate, is partially converted to alpha limit dextrins, maltose and glucose in the mouth by enzymes in saliva, and these sugars are then available for metabolising into acids by plaque bacteria. However for starch rich staple foods such as bread, potatoes and rice the rate of conversion is slow and dietary starch by itself is very much less important than dietary sugars as a cause of dental caries. Raw starch, such as found in fruits and vegetables, is virtually non-cariogenic. Research conducted in the UK during World War II showed that while starch consumption increased and sugars consumption decreased caries prevalence decreased despite the increase in starch consumption. Recent research has shown that when starch is cooked at very high temperatures, such as for the production of some snack foods including biscuits and cakes, then the conversion to glucose in the mouth can occur more rapidly.

From a theoretical aspect, sugar-free chewing gum may have a positive benefit for dental health by increasing salivary flow during chewing, which helps to neutralise plaque acid activity. The majority of clinical studies have found a positive benefit.

Table 1 Cariogenic sugars	
Sugars and other compounds added to food and drinks during processing, manufacture or before consumption as sweeteners and that have the potential to cause dental caries.	
glucose*	maltose
fructose*	glucose syrup
hydrolysed starch	maltodextrins
sucrose*	oligofructose
invert sugar	corn syrup

*non-cariogenic when contained in the whole fresh fruits, vegetables and grains.

Table 2 Products that are essentially a mixture of sugars	
brown sugar (mainly sucrose)	treacle
maple syrup	honey
golden syrup	

Table 3 Non-cariogenic sweeteners	
Bulk sweeteners mainly used to add sweetness, calories and bulk to confectionery products.	
maltitol syrup	lactitol
mannitol	xylitol
isomalt	maltitol
sorbitol	

Xylitol

There is evidence from laboratory and clinical studies that xylitol is not only non-cariogenic, but may also suppress the growth of some acidogenic bacteria in plaque. There is some evidence that the beneficial effect on the plaque bacteria may be passed from a mother to her children. The use of xylitol in chewing gum has been the subject of a number of extensive clinical trials, the majority of which have shown a significant caries-inhibiting effect however the evidence is not conclusive [30]. If consumed in excess, bulk sweeteners can have a laxative effect. While overt diarrhoea is a rare side-effect, children are at greater risk. There is a statutory requirement in the UK for these sweeteners to carry the labeling that excessive consumption may produce laxative effects.

Table 4 Intense sweeteners added in small amounts often to soft drinks	
Acesulfame K	Aspartame
Saccharin	Cyclamate
Thaumatin	Sucralose
Neohesperidine DC	

Combinations of sugars and intense sweeteners such as saccharin are used in some products; however the latter will not have a protective role and such products must be classified as cariogenic. Concentrated soft drinks, which are the main source of artificial sweeteners in the diet of young children, should be diluted with extra water for these young consumers to avoid excessive intake. It is advised that ideally drinks containing artificial sweeteners such as aspartame or saccharin should not be given to young children. If they are given they should be diluted with at least 10 parts water to one part concentrate. Even if well diluted, such drinks are acidic and have the potential to cause erosion (see chapter 6).

It must be remembered that manufacturing problems related to sugars substitution are not just limited to sweetness, cost and safety. Sugars give bulk to many foods and influence properties such as viscosity, texture and shelf life.

The pattern of sugar intake

After consuming sugar, acid is rapidly generated in the dental plaque and, within 1–2 minutes, plaque pH has fallen to levels that favour enamel demineralisation. The return to neutrality takes between 20 minutes and two hours, depending on such factors as salivary flow rate and buffering capacity as well as plaque thickness and composition. Maximum acid production is achieved by modest sugar concentrations, beyond which increased concentrations do not give a greater fall in pH. However, frequent sugar intakes will not allow time for the pH to recover and will prolong the period of plaque acidity. This pattern may allow demineralisation to exceed remineralisation resulting in a progressive loss of minerals from enamel as illustrated in Figure 2.4. These observations are supported by animal experiments that have shown a direct correlation between sucrose frequency and caries levels. It has been shown that, in human volunteers who stopped toothbrushing and used two-hourly sucrose rinses, enamel demineralisation occurred within three weeks. However, as the amount of NMES consumed has been shown to be independently related to caries experience and as frequency and amount are strongly linked, advice must be to reduce both. This advice is supported by a report from the UK Committee on Medical Aspects of Food Policy (Dietary Sugars and Human Disease 1989) [28].

The frequency and time of consumption of sugars-sweetened foods and drinks have both been shown to be important factors in determining caries levels. Sugars consumed with main meals appear to be of less significance because they are cleared from the mouth by other foods together with the high salivary flow rate generated by eating. Other foods taken as part of the meal, such as cheese, may help stimulate salivary flow and raise the calcium level in plaque so that remineralisation is promoted. However, sugars-sweetened items consumed between meals appear to have a much more detrimental effect. The World Health Organisation has recommended a population target for the amount of "free sugars" consumed: these sugars should contribute no more than a maximum of 10% of energy intake. In addition, a target for the frequency of consumption of foods and/or drinks containing "free sugars" has been set at a maximum of four times per day and there is some evidence to support this recommendation. (these recommendations are under periodic review). In England the Scientific Advisory Committee on Nutrition provides recommendations on limiting dietary sugars intake (www.sacn.gov.uk/). While this advice provides a pragmatic guide for individuals, there is no completely safe frequency of consumption because of factors such as variations in the nature and composition of saliva, the pattern and time of consumption of the sugars and the nature of the sugar item itself [31].

Research has confirmed that bedtime is the worst time to consume a sugars-sweetened drink or snack. This is due to the low salivary flow rate during sleep and to the fact that toothbrushing is unlikely to remove all traces of any sugary snack taken before bed. Children who consumed both a sugary drink and snack in the hour before bed were found to have four times the number of decayed teeth compared to children who had neither [32]. However, one of the benefits of low salivary flow at night time does mean that when the teeth are brushed with a fluoridated toothpaste, the fluoride will remain in the mouth for a prolonged time and will not be cleared so quickly by the saliva. Sugars in medicines can also cause decay. Many paediatric medicines, including those sold without prescription, have sugar-free alternatives. Clinicians should prescribe sugar-free medicines and parents/carers should request them. Pharmacists should be encouraged to stock and recommend sugar-free alternatives to the most commonly used prescription and general sale medicines.

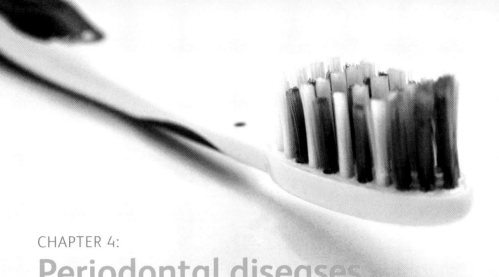

CHAPTER 4

Periodontal diseases

Key points

- The risk of developing periodontal disease can be reduced by careful and effective daily toothbrushing.
  Evidence Base A

- The risk of developing periodontal disease can be reduced by not smoking.
  Evidence Base A

Periodontal diseases

While there are many diseases, both acute and chronic, that affect the gums and the surrounding bone and fibres that support the teeth, by far the most common are gingivitis and chronic periodontitis. Gingivitis can begin as early as childhood and presents as inflammation of the gum margin, with redness, swelling and bleeding on brushing (Fig. 4.1). Gingivitis can be reversed by effective oral hygiene. Without adequate personal oral care, a second stage, termed chronic periodontitis can occur (often referred to simply as 'periodontitis'). In this stage, which can begin as early as adolescence, the bone and fibres that support the teeth are progressively destroyed (Fig. 4.2). However, the rate of destruction can vary greatly both between and within individuals and is dependent on local factors within the mouth and on host susceptibility due to systemic factors such as smoking and diabetes. Loss of supporting bone may lead eventually to loosening and finally loss of the tooth, although the process can be slowed or stopped from progressing further by a combination of personal care and professional treatment.

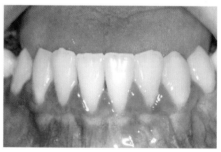

Fig. 4.1   Gingivitis.

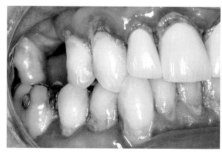

Fig. 4.2   Periodontitis

Cause

Periodontitis is initiated by dental plaque – a soft, sticky film composed mainly of bacteria, which forms on the teeth and is present in all mouths. Poor oral hygiene allows plaque to accumulate, especially at the necks of the teeth and between them. However, it is the host response to plaque that determines the rate and severity of disease progression. The response of the body to any insult, be it physical or induced by microorganisms, is by inflammation. The nature of the inflammatory response is determined by many factors, including the extrinsic nature of whatever is inducing the inflammatory response as well as intrinsic factors such as the nature of the immune and inflammatory response to the insult (which can vary both between individuals and also within an individual over time), and the presence of conditions that compromise or alter the inflammatory response such as smoking or diabetes.

In any inflammatory condition, the outcome is dependent on the balance between the severity of the insult that provokes the inflammation and the host's response. In periodontal disease, it is the failure of the inflammatory response to effectively overcome the challenge and maintain the health of the fibres and bone supporting the teeth that prolongs the inflammatory state and leads to the progressive destruction that we see in periodontal disease. The subsequent progressive destruction appears dependent upon a complex plaque–host relationship that is still being investigated. Important risk factors in this relationship include diabetes and smoking.

Diabetes, obesity and periodontal disease

The global rise of obesity, both adult and childhood, is leading to an increasing prevalence of diabetes, cardiovascular disease and cancers, a trend likely to continue for at least the next two decades. Diabetes was estimated to affect about 250 million people worldwide in 2007, a figure predicted to rise to 350 million by 2030. It has been estimated that obese persons have a more than ten-fold increased risk of developing type 2 diabetes compared with normal-weight persons. There is now a considerable evidence establishing diabetes as a risk factor for chronic periodontitis, especially where glycaemic control is poor, and the increased risk has been estimated at three-fold. This appears to be true also for type 1 diabetes and there is evidence for increased risk of periodontitis in affected children.

While it is accepted that both type 1 and type 2 diabetes are important risk factors for the development and progression of periodontitis, there is growing evidence that obesity is both an indirect risk factor, because it affects glycaemic control, and a direct risk factor because secretion of pro-inflammatory mediators by adipose tissue modifies the periodontal reaction to the plaque.

It is established that periodontal disease can adversely affect glycaemic control in people with diabetes and that glycaemic control can be improved by effective periodontal treatment, thereby reducing the risk of diabetes co-morbidity. Thus there is a two-way relationship between the two conditions, with diabetes increasing the risk and severity of periodontal disease and treatment for the disease aiding diabetes control[33]. Dental professionals should recognise these interlinked risk factors, include an assessment of diabetes status for all patients and, when periodontitis is diagnosed, treat effectively and work in collaboration with medical practitioners to help improve both oral and general health [34]. They should also be aware of the signs of undiagnosed diabetes in their patients, such as periodontal disease in the absence of local factors, as well as fatigue, thirst and weight loss and advise such patients to seek appropriate medical investigation[35].

Plaque retention factors

Any irregularity around the teeth will encourage the accumulation of plaque by making tooth cleaning difficult. Such factors include crooked teeth,

overhanging edges on fillings, poorly contoured fillings, some types of partial dentures and calculus. Calculus (often referred to as 'tartar') is plaque which has become calcified and hardened. Calculus is a plaque-retentive feature and renders effective oral hygiene more difficult. Calculus can form above the gum line (supragingival) and below the gum margin (subgingival). As periodontal disease progresses, the shallow space between the gum margin and the tooth (the sulcus or gingival crevice) deepens to form a periodontal pocket in which plaque and subgingival calculus accumulate, and which is more difficult to keep clean.

Risk factors

There is a strong association between the amount of plaque accumulation and the reaction of the oral tissues. However, variations are seen both in the inflammatory response in the periodontal tissues and the rate of destruction of the supporting bone. This may be due to a number of factors. The types of bacteria present in plaque vary both between individuals and at different sites within an individual mouth. There is very strong evidence that smoking increases the risk of periodontitis and reduces the effectiveness of treatment[36]. This very important risk factor should be emphasised to all smokers. People with diabetes, especially if glycaemic control is poor, are at increased risk as explained above. In many cases, however, the cause of variation in susceptibility to periodontitis is likely to result from differences between individuals in terms of the inflammatory response to the long-term presence of the subgingival biofilm (plaque) with exaggerated and prolonged inflammation being a major cause of tissue destruction. Moreover, failure of inflammation-resolving mechanisms in some patients appears to cause the initially defensive acute inflammatory response to be replaced by a destructive chronic inflammation.

The gum margin around the necks of the teeth is a unique structure in the body as it is an imperfect junction between two quite different body tissues; hard, calcified tooth surface and the soft, vascular tissue of the gums. The body's immune and inflammatory defense system has to fight a constant battle to prevent harmful bacteria from penetrating this junction and anything that affects this defense system can produce a reaction at the gum margin, usually inflammation. This was first seen as scurvy in seamen before the need for vitamin C was recognised. However, today, a common example is the change produced by the hormonal disturbance during pregnancy, where even modest deposits of plaque can sometimes produce a pronounced inflammatory gingival condition known as pregnancy gingivitis. However, mothers should be assured that pregnancy itself does not cause periodontal disease. While pregnancy gingivitis may resolve after birth of the child, pre-existing chronic periodontal disease will not, and professional help is required. Other systemic conditions that can cause gingival change, often as a first indication, include anaemia, diabetes and leukaemia.

Prevention

In most cases gingivitis precedes chronic periodontitis. The main strategy for limiting periodontitis is by plaque control directed to maintaining gingival and periodontal health. This must be considered at two levels – what people can do for themselves by way of plaque control on a daily basis, and what dentists and hygienists/therapists can do to eliminate plaque retention factors and to advise the individual on the most appropriate home care.

What people can do for themselves:

The most important plaque control method is effective toothbrushing with a fluoride toothpaste and it should be established as a daily routine from the time of tooth eruption. Toothbrushing skills should be taught to people of all ages. The precise technique is less important than the result, which is that plaque is removed effectively and daily without causing damage to the teeth or gums.

A gentle scrub technique is effective for most people and is easy to teach and is readily accepted. Careful use of this method with a recommended type of brush should be taught as it can provide effective plaque removal, but the use of only very gentle pressure and a soft toothbrush should be emphasised (see Chapter 5). Most authorities recommend a brush with a small head bearing densely packed soft to medium synthetic filaments. Incorrect toothbrushing techniques involving excessive pressure may considerably increase gum recession and loss of tooth substance by mechanical abrasion and should therefore be corrected (see Fig 4.3). The use of dental floss as an aid to plaque removal has not been unequivocally established as being effective in controlling periodontal inflammation. However mini-interdental "bottle" type brushes that are used for cleaning between teeth are of established value and easy to use where there is sufficient space between the teeth. Their use should be encouraged by dental professionals for plaque control but they must be employed correctly and require professional advice and instruction[37].

Plaque-disclosing agents, which stain plaque to make it easily visible can be a useful aid to improving plaque control. They will not in themselves remove plaque, but will show areas where plaque remains after brushing.

An additional method of plaque control is the use of antiseptics, of which chlorhexidine is the most effective. Although this antiseptic is on general sale in the UK in mouthrinse and gel forms, its tendency to stain teeth and impair taste makes it generally unacceptable for long-term use and it is only advised for use up to one month. Many popular toothpastes contain other chemical plaque-suppressing agents such as zinc salts and triclosan, although triclosan has been associated with some environmental concerns. While these agents are less effective than chlorhexidine, they have been shown to be of some value to gingival health.

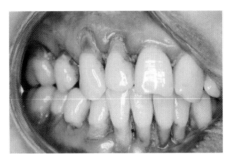

Fig. 4.3   Toothbrush abrasion

What dental professionals can do:

It is the responsibility of the dentist to ensure that any treatment provided minimises plaque retention; this is a part of treatment planning. Clear advice must also be given on the need to clean bridges, dentures and orthodontic appliances (braces) effectively and regularly. Calculus that forms on the teeth above the gum level and below the gum level within the pockets encourages plaque accumulation; this should be removed regularly by careful professional treatment. The most appropriate non-surgical treatment strategy for periodontal diseases is referred to as root surface debridement and is commonly and efficiently undertaken with ultrasonic instruments and area-specific curettes; the focus of the treatment is to disrupt and reduce the plaque biofilm and remove calculus without damaging the root surface or attempting to purposefully remove cementum. However, the most important role of the professional in treating periodontitis is to instil a need for behavioural or life-style change aimed at improving and maintaining oral health through effective daily oral hygiene using an effective and atraumatic toothbrushing technique and instruction on the use of mini-interdental brushes where appropriate. This should be underpinned by a clear understanding of the cause of periodontitis, with emphasis on the identification (and where possible, elimination) of any specific risk factors such as smoking and poor glycaemic control in patients with diabetes and appropriate support and monitoring in conjunction with the patient's medical practitioner. Guidance on the provision of smoking cessation advice is given in Appendix 1. Other, more complex interventions for the prevention and treatment of periodontitis are available, but are beyond the scope of this book. More information on plaque control can be found in Chapter 5.

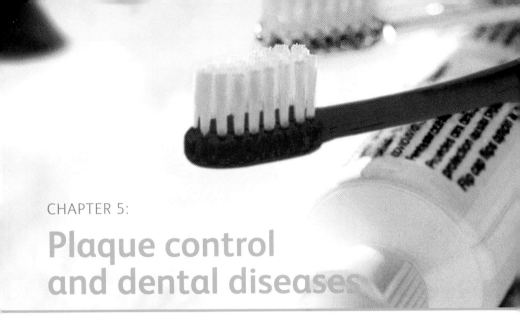

CHAPTER 5:

Plaque control and dental diseases

Key points

- Twice-daily brushing with a manual or powered toothbrush and a fluoride-containing toothpaste is the principal means of plaque control.
  Evidence Base A

- Other aids such as interdental (bottle type) brushes can be effective but are best used following professional advice.
  Evidence Base C

Plaque and dental diseases

There is ample evidence of an association between plaque and periodontitis in children and adults. Plaque deposits have been shown to cause gingival inflammation, which is reversed by plaque removal. It follows that plaque control can be endorsed for the prevention of gingivitis, although it should be remembered that once the bone and fibres supporting the tooth have been lost as a result of chronic periodontitis, then plaque control alone is probably insufficient to stabilise the condition. A combination of personal plaque control and professional treatment may then be needed to prevent further bone loss.

Based on clinical observation, it had been suggested that dental caries could be controlled by highly effective toothbrushing, without the benefit of fluoride toothpaste. Some research studies have shown that highly efficient toothbrushing techniques can reduce caries. However, plaque removal by normal toothbrushing alone does not appear to be as effective, as some plaque is left in fissures and other stagnation sites where caries occurs, and plaque rapidly begins to reform on cleaned tooth surfaces. For caries prevention, the real value of toothbrushing is now thought to be that it combines plaque removal with the application of fluoride to the tooth surface.

Plaque removal for children

It is generally agreed that most children have insufficient manual dexterity to achieve effective plaque removal with a toothbrush until at least six to seven years of age, or until the time when they can use cutlery to feed themselves with proficiency. Parents should be advised to brush their children's teeth thoroughly twice a day using a small brush. One method of toothbrushing is for the parent to stand behind the child and tilt the child's head upwards so that all tooth surfaces can be brushed using a gentle scrub motion.

Plaque removal for adults

The gentle horizontal scrub method of toothbrushing is effective in plaque removal and is easily taught and accepted. However it is essential that the use of this simple technique does not abrade the teeth or gums. It should be carried out with a small toothbrush for ease of access. Holding the brush with the fingers in a 'pen' grip may avoid excessive force. Therefore, the toothbrush should be held with a finger grip similar to the way one holds a pencil, not a fist grip. The method is to place the filaments of the brush at the neck of the tooth and to use very short horizontal movements to dislodge plaque from the stagnation areas at the gum margins around the teeth. The biting surfaces of side and back teeth should then be brushed. Emphasis should be placed on small forward and backwards movements and gentle pressure, together with an unhurried systematic approach to the cleaning of all surfaces. Other techniques that are just as effective at plaque removal and less traumatic to the tissues are the roll, modified bass (which is the main technique taught in undergraduate schools in the UK) and the modified Stillman technique. A vigorous horizontal "scrubbing" motion should be avoided as this can cause wear at the necks of the teeth leading to the formation of "V" shaped toothbrush abrasion grooves, especially if combined with the use of a hard brush and an abrasive smokers-type toothpaste.

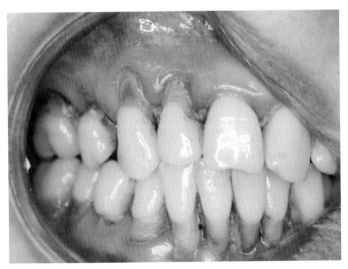

Fig 5.1   Toothbrush abrasion grooves.

The use of dental floss as an aid to plaque removal has not been unequivocally established as being effective in controlling periodontal inflammation. However mini-interdental "bottle" type brushes that are used for cleaning between teeth are of established value and easy to use where there is sufficient space between the teeth[37]. Their use should be encouraged as an interdental cleaning aid in addition to, and not instead of effective and atraumatic toothbrushing.

Recommended toothbrush specifications

While there is a wide variation in toothbrush design, little evidence exists to support specific recommendations. The size of the toothbrush head should be appropriate to the user but it should be remembered that a smaller head will give better access to the back of the mouth and those tooth surfaces that a large-headed brush cannot reach. The filaments (bristles) should be of a synthetic material, round-ended and of a soft to medium texture (ISO 20126: 2012). For children or adults with limited manual dexterity, it can be an advantage to choose a toothbrush with a large handle that provides a firm, comfortable grip. When the bristles become deformed or splayed, plaque removal becomes less effective and the toothbrush should be replaced.

Powered toothbrushes

Modern powered toothbrushes have become very popular. Several independent systematic reviews of existing studies concluded that powered toothbrushes are at least as effective as manual toothbrushes and there is no evidence that they will cause more injuries to the gums than manual brushes . Powered toothbrushes with a rotation oscillation action (i.e. the head rotates in one direction and then the other) or ultrasonic vibration appear to be slightly better at removing plaque and reducing gum inflammation than manual toothbrushes, but the long-term benefits are unclear[38]. Some individuals like the 'feel' of powered toothbrushes and they can be helpful in those with limited manual dexterity, such as arthritis sufferers; furthermore, the novelty value in children can encourage compliance with their brushing regime. As with manual toothbrushes, the heads do wear out and need to be replaced regularly.

Chemical plaque suppressants

Of the many agents that have been tested, chlorhexidine gluconate has proved to be the most effective plaque suppressant under clinical conditions. Chlorhexidine is on general sale in the UK in mouthrinse, gel and spray forms. Chlorhexidine can cause staining of teeth, which is difficult to remove from white fillings, and can impair taste. While clinical experience in daily sustained use is limited, two years being the duration of the longest clinical trial reported to date, no other major adverse effects have been reported from oral use. Nevertheless, it is generally unacceptable for long-term unsupervised use, one month being the normal limit. It can be of value for short-term use when toothbrushing is difficult or painful, but works best on clean teeth by inhibiting plaque formation. While in worldwide use for many years as a general purpose antiseptic, chlorhexidine has been associated with severe allergic reactions in a small number of reported cases.

Other antiseptics without the adverse effects of chlorhexidine are used in many mouthrinses and toothpastes. These include the phenol derivative, triclosan, and zinc compounds and some essential oils. Use of such products may provide limited benefits to plaque control and gingival health. There is evidence that the non-cariogenic sweetener xylitol inhibits the growth of some plaque bacteria (see Chapter 3). However, its value for the prevention of periodontitis has not been established.

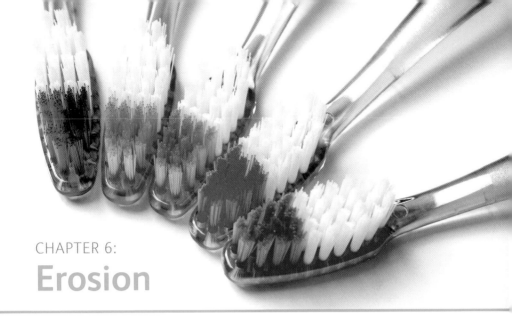

CHAPTER 6

Erosion

Key points

- Limit the frequency of intake of acidic beverages.
  Evidence Base B

- Avoid brushing for one hour after an 'acidic episode'.
  Evidence Base C

What is erosion?

Erosion is the loss of tooth substance caused by the direct action of chemicals on the tooth surface. It is quite different from caries in both appearance and causation. While erosion can occur by chemical action alone, it is sometimes linked to both attrition of the teeth due to grinding them, often at night, or eating coarse foods and with abrasion due to excessive brushing with a hard brush or an abrasive toothpaste. Erosion is therefore classed as a type of tooth wear. Indeed, tooth wear in many individuals is due to a combination of attrition, abrasion and erosion in differing proportions.

Clinical presentation

Erosion was described as early as 1892 among Sicilian lemon pickers. The characteristic appearance is loss of enamel and in more severe cases of dentine from specific sites. Erosion should not be confused with dental caries. While caries affects the surfaces of the teeth where plaque stagnates, erosion affects plaque- free surfaces. Primarily, these are the palatal (inside) aspects of the upper front teeth followed by the labial (lip) aspects of these teeth and the occlusal (biting) surfaces of the premolar (side) and molar (back) teeth (Fig. 6.1). In the primary dentition the incisal (biting) edges of the upper front teeth are often lost first (Fig. 6.2). In the early stages pain is not a feature, but as enamel loss progresses, especially if this is rapid, sensitivity to thermal change and acidic drinks becomes established and more persistent pain can occur in severe cases.

Cause

Erosion is usually due to acids entering the mouth. Gastric reflux brings acid into the mouth and is thought to affect up to 70% of individuals at some time. Causes include hiatus hernia, pregnancy, motion sickness, alcoholism, obesity and eating disorders, of which it can be an early sign. However, dietary factors are thought to be the most common cause today. While citrus fruits have erosive potential, there is little evidence to link the consumption of whole fruit with increased erosion in a normal population probably because of the saliva-stimulating effect of chewing. In contrast, fruit juice is erosive and the frequent consumption of juices has been linked in many reports to increased tooth wear. Possibly of greater significance is the erosive potential of soft drinks, including carbonated and fruit-based ones as well as sports-type drinks. The rapid rise in consumption of fruit juice and soft drinks, following the development of modern containers such as the tetrapak, plastic bottles and aluminum cans, has been blamed for what is generally perceived as an increase in the prevalence of erosion, especially among youngsters. The relationship between frequency of consumption of such drinks and erosion is now established[39].

The principal ingredient linked to erosion is citric acid, which is found in most fruit juices and soft drinks, however other fruit acids may have an effect. The erosive effect is partly due to its low pH and also because it can demineralise enamel by binding to calcium and removing it from the tooth surface, a process called chelation. Cola-type drinks may also contain phosphoric acid, which produces a low pH. The recent popularity of "alcopop" type drinks, which are fruit-flavoured alcoholic beverages, strong ciders and sports drinks, all of which have a low pH, has caused concern, but as yet no substantive evidence is available. The same is true of "fruit smoothies" which are blends of fruit and fruit juice and have been shown in laboratory studies to be erosive. While the pH of a drink is an indicator of its erosive potential, a measure called total titratable acidity, which gives the capacity of a liquid to dissolve mineral, is a better guide.

Some other factors are important in determining the risk of erosion. These include the flow rate and buffering capacity of saliva, the manner and frequency of consumption of erosive drinks and the consumption of other foods such as cheese and milk. There is anecdotal evidence that the common habit of swishing carbonated drinks around the mouth before swallowing may increase the danger. In addition, acidic ice lollipops and acid-based sweets may have erosive potential.

Although the Basic Erosive Wear Examination is becoming established, there is a lack of a universally accepted index for the assessment of erosion, either prevalence or incidence and consequently there are no reliable long-term data to indicate changes in the prevalence of erosion over time[40]. Most clinicians believe that prevalence has increased during the later part of the last century. From the many studies in the literature the prevalence of enamel erosion in children appears to vary from less than 10% to 80% according to age. For erosion into dentine the figures are lower, but may affect 25% of children with primary teeth[41]. The higher levels usually found in the primary dentition are thought to be due to the practice of giving fruit juice in feeding bottles or feeder cups.

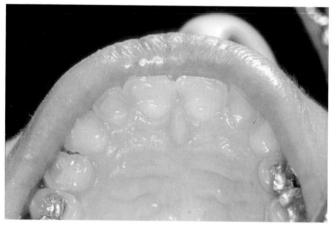

Fig. 6.1   Dental erosion on the palatal aspect of upper anterior teeth. Almost all of the enamel has been lost.

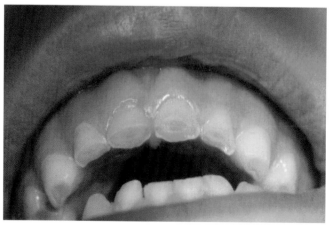

Fig. 6.2 Dental erosion of deciduous teeth.

Prevention

The currently available preventive advice relies upon expert consensus and best practice, however it is generally agreed that erosion can be prevented by reducing the intake of erosive drinks and food. While no safe limit can be established, any reduction is desirable. Children and young adults especially should not have acidic beverages as their main fluid intake. Fresh fruit is a really important part of the diet, however frequent consumption between meals, as with the Sicilian lemon pickers, should be avoided as the sugar and acids in some fruit can damage the teeth if eaten too often. The practices of swishing and frequent sipping of acidic drinks should be discouraged. Taking milk or cheese after such foods or drinks may be beneficial. Drinking erosive beverages through a straw has been shown to help, but only if the tip is placed well back in the mouth. It is also sensible to avoid toothbrushing for a period of time after an erosive episode as the brush can damage the softened enamel. There is no conclusive evidence as to how long this should be, but a period of one hour is accepted by most experts.

The resistance of the teeth to erosion can be increased by the use of topical fluorides. Whilst twice daily use of a fluoride toothpaste is considered essential, mouthrinses are also of value. Fluoride mouthrinses should not be used by children under 6 years of age. The professional application of fluoride varnishes and gels can give added benefit, both by increasing enamel acid resistance and in reducing sensitivity. The degree of protection given by these various topical measures is still being investigated. In severe cases some form of restoration is usually necessary, often crowns for permanent teeth. Where gastric regurgitation is suspected because of physical or emotional problems such as in eating disorders, the patient should be advised to consult their medical practitioner.

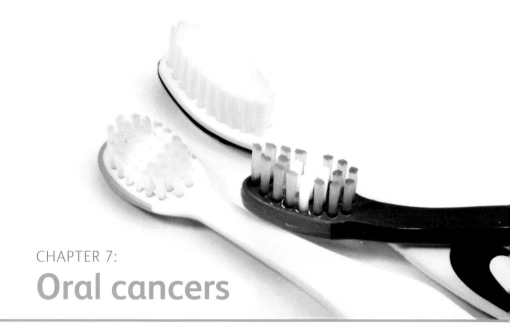

CHAPTER 7

Oral cancers

Key points

- Smoking, other forms of tobacco use and frequent alcohol consumption are the main risk factors, especially in combination.
  Evidence Base A

- White or red patches and oral ulceration present for more than three weeks require immediate investigation.
  Evidence Base C

- Smokers who wish to give up should be given appropriate support to do so.
  Evidence Base C

Oral tumours

As elsewhere in the body, both benign and malignant tumours can occur in the mouth. Benign tumours tend to be slow growing and localised and are rarely life-threatening. However, malignant tumours can grow rapidly, infiltrate the surrounding area and spread to the lymph nodes or to other parts of the body, with the formation of secondary or metastatic deposits, especially in the bones, lungs or other organs. If detected early, when the lesions are small, and treated, a complete cure is often possible, but delay makes treatment difficult and approximately half of all cases prove fatal within five years.

Squamous cell carcinoma

The most common type of oral cancer is squamous cell carcinoma, which accounts for about 90% of all oral malignancies. They arise from the oral mucosa lining the mouth and covering the tongue. In the majority of cases squamous cell carcinomas present late as an ulcer, most commonly in the floor of the mouth, the lateral border of the tongue, or inside the lips. Carcinomas may also arise within a pre-existing white, red, or thickened area of mucosa and at the earliest stage may not show obvious signs of ulceration but are usually red or speckled. Thickened white areas of mucosa, termed leukoplakia, are well recognised as potential sites for malignant change and the appearance of red spots or ulceration within a leukoplakia is often an indication of this change (Fig. 7.1). It has been estimated that up to 17% of leukoplakias will undergo malignant change.

Malignant ulcers differ from other innocent ulcers by persisting for more than two weeks after any cause is removed. Unlike other forms of oral ulceration, they do not heal or resolve spontaneously. Indeed, any ulcer present for more than three weeks must be investigated without delay by referral to a specialist.

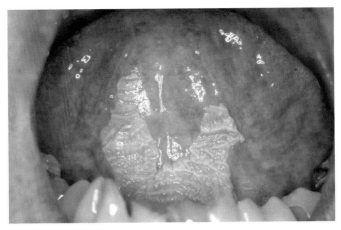

Fig. 7.1   Leukoplakia on the ventral (under) surface
of the tongue.

Other oral tumours

Other tumours can arise in or around the mouth, such as within the jaw
bones or from salivary glands, connective tissue, blood vessels or nerves.
These tumours generally present as swellings, but in some cases the first
signs may be loosening of teeth, spontaneous fracture of the jaw or
enlargement of the lymph nodes in the neck.

Prevalence and prognosis

Globally, cancers of the lip and oral cavity account for 2% of all cancers with
an estimated 263,000 cases in 2008, but they are the second most common
cancer in males and the fourth most common cancer in females in South-
Central Asia, accounting for 7% of the total cancers diagnosed in this region
in 2008. Tobacco and betel chewing explains the high incidence in some
developing countries, whereas tobacco smoking and alcohol consumption
are the major causes of oral cancer in developed countries. In the UK it is
estimated that there were over 6500 new cases in 2010, an increase of 26%
in males and 30% in females, since 2000 and responsible for about 1,700
deaths. The incidence is more than twice that of cervical cancer. Almost
twice as many males are affected as females and the greatest increase in
recent years has been for men in their 40s and 50s. For oral cancers detected

at the earliest stage, the five-year survival rate is about 90%, but this falls to about 20% for those presenting at the latest stage[42]. The poor, overall five-year survival rate is thought to be due to the late presentation of many cases. This finding is even more distressing because the mouth is the easiest body cavity to examine. While most cases occur in men, and many cases occur in the over 60s, in recent years there has been a shift towards an earlier age of onset (45-59 years) and an increase in the number of women affected.

Cause and prevention

The main risk factors for oral cancers are tobacco or alcohol and a combination of these factors appears to multiply the risk[43]. While a recent meta-analysis of published data has found that, on average, current cigarette smokers have a three-fold increased risk of oral cancer, the relative risk for long-term smokers who also consume alcohol may be over 35 times greater than non-smokers who are infrequent drinkers[44]. The risk of oral cancer associated with smoking is both dose and duration dependent and while smoking cessation leads to a fall in risk and about 50% of leukoplakias (see Chapter 8) appear to resolve, a recent study showed that it takes 20 years or longer for the risk to reduce to that of those who have never smoked. Another recent study estimated that around 70% of oral and pharyngeal cancers in men and around 55% in women in the UK in 2010 were caused by smoking tobacco. As with other cancers, "passive smoking", the exposure to secondhand smoke, may increase oral cancer risk, one study showing a 63% increase for never smokers exposed at home or at work, increasing to 84% for those exposed for more than 15 years. The use of smokeless tobacco has also been implicated as a risk factor. The habits of chewing tobacco and reverse smoking (with the lit end inside the mouth) have been found to be linked to high rates of oral cancer, while the common practice amongst some Asian communities of chewing "betel nut quid", "paan" or "ghutka", an addictive blend of tobacco and other vegetable matter, is linked to the high prevalence of oral cancers in the Indian sub-continent and Asian communities in other parts of the world.

Alcohol is a major risk factor for oral cancers and it has been estimated that in 2010 in the UK around 37% of oral and pharyngeal cancers in men and 17% in women were linked to alcohol consumption. For an alcohol intake of 25 grams (3 units)/day, risk increases by 80%, and there is a three-fold risk increase for 50 grams (6 units)/day and a six-fold risk increase for 100 grams (12 units)/day. The risk is greater in smokers than non-smokers, with a six-fold risk increase for heavy drinking by smokers, compared with a three-fold risk increase for non or ex- smokers. Heavy drinkers and smokers may have more than 35 times the risk compared to those who abstain from both. In the UK, consumption of alcohol has more than doubled since the 1950s, from 3.9 to 8.6 litres of pure alcohol per head per year and this may partly explain the worrying increase in the incidence of oral cancers [44]. Concerns have been expressed about the potential risks of using alcohol containing mouthwashes, but there is no evidence that use of an alcohol containing rinse increases the risk of oral cancers. Nevertheless there is a hypothetical risk and the increasing availability of alcohol free mouthwashes suggests that it may be prudent to advise patients to use these[45].

Other risk factors include a family history of head and neck cancers, pre-existing white patches on the oral mucosa, including those related to candida infection (see Chapter 8), some viral infections and immuno-suppressive treatment for conditions such as HIV and AIDS.

There is emerging evidence concerning the human papilloma virus (HPV) of which there are over 100 strains and is now the main sexually transmitted infection in the USA. While recognised as a major cause of cervical cancers, there is now clear evidence that HPV infection with virus strains 16 and 18 is linked to 90% of cases of squamous carcinoma of the oropharynx (posterior tongue and tonsils) and may be responsible for the rapidly increasing prevalence of such cancers in younger individuals who do not smoke or drink, but probably associated with oral sex practices[46]. HPV linked oropharyngeal tumours appear to be a distinct sub-group however overall HPV is at present a minor cause of oral cancers and has not yet been implicated in lesions towards the anterior aspect of the mouth. In many developed countries including the UK, most EU countries and the USA, vaccination against the main strains has been implemented as a public health measure for young girls, yet there is a persuasive argument for the vaccination of boys and this policy has been implemented in Australia, Canada and the USA[47].

There is evidence that the prevention of many types of malignancy benefit from a higher intake of fresh fruit and vegetables, resulting from their content of vitamin and anti-oxidant compounds. Overall however the most important approach for reducing mortality and morbidity from oral cancers is early diagnosis and this argues the case for regular whole mouth examinations and immediate referral of suspicious lesions to an appropriate secondary care clinician. Surgery and radiotherapy for head and neck cancers can result in major facial and oral deformities and reduced salivary flow. Loss of teeth and a dry mouth can lead to significant dental problems and carefully planned and integrated care is needed.

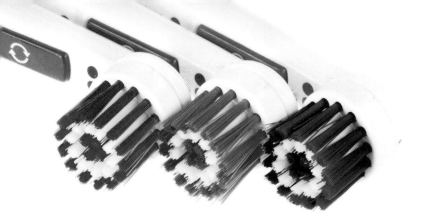

CHAPTER 8:
Other oral diseases

Key points

- Oral candidosis, when not associated with dentures, may be a sign of systemic disease causing immunosuppression. Evidence Base B

- Dentures should be removed and cleaned every night and should be replaced when damaged, ill-fitting or worn out. Evidence Base B

Oral candidosis

While the fungus Candida albicans is present in most mouths, in some circumstances excessive multiplication can present as various forms of both acute and chronic inflammation. The most common presentations are angular chelitis, a chronic infection of the angles of the mouth, usually seen in older people, especially those with old, worn dentures (Fig. 8.1) and denture sore mouth, (the term is a misnomer – as the mouth is not usually sore) a chronic, generally painless infection, usually seen in the palate where a denture is worn at night, instead of being removed as generally advised (Fig. 8.2). Some cases are associated with poor nutrition, chronic anaemia, diabetes or depression of the immune system as in HIV and AIDS infection. Prevention of these common forms depends on treating any systemic factors and the removal and thorough cleaning of dentures each night as well as their replacement when they are worn out (see Chapter 10).

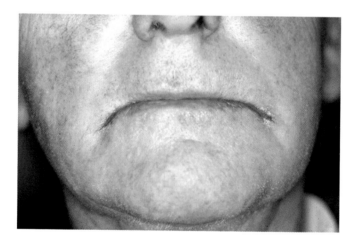

Fig. 8.1 Angular chelitis, a form of chronic Candida infection.

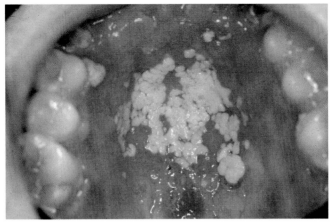

Fig. 8.2   Candida infection in the palate associated with poor hygiene practice in the wearing of a partial upper denture. The yellow clumps are colonies of Candida organisms growing on the mucosa.

Oral ulceration

About 25% of the population suffers from minor apthous ulceration – the common mouth ulcer – on a regular basis. The ulcers occur either singly or in small crops, often inside the lips or cheek and heal with or without treatment within 10 days. The cause remains unknown, although some cases are associated with systemic illness such as anaemia or diabetes. A more severe form, major apthous ulceration, generally produces solitary ulcers, which take up to a month to heal, often leaving a residual scar. Herpes simplex infection can cause a common form of oral ulceration. Viral in origin, it can produce a very sore mouth with crops of small grey ulcers that generally heal spontaneously within 10 days. The primary infection can occur in infancy and may be confused with teething. When young children are affected, they can become rapidly dehydrated and an adequate fluid intake is essential. As the virus often remains dormant in the tissues, secondary attacks can occur, either in the mouth or on the lips as herpes labalis or cold sores.

Ulceration can also be caused by trauma, such as lip biting (sometimes with self-injurious behaviour) or by the sharp edge of a denture, however all innocent ulcers should heal within a month.

White and red patches

A number of conditions can present as white or red patches in the mouth. Some patches can be caused by simple friction from cheek biting, but others may be forms of chronic candidosis or premalignant conditions (see chapter 7). Any white or red patch persisting for more than three weeks must be investigated without delay.

Dry mouth

Xerostomia, or dry mouth, is a common condition that can make eating or even speech difficult and can increase the risk of dental caries. Although it can affect people of all ages, it appears to be more common in older people. However, recent research suggests that age, in itself, is not an important factor, but rather, it may be as a consequence of the wide range of drugs that induce xerostomia as a side-effect and which many elderly people require. Specific causes of xerostomia include diabetes, a blocked salivary duct, chronic dehydration and more rarely, a salivary gland tumour or Sjögrens syndrome. A very severe form of xerostomia can follow from radiotherapy for tumours of the head or neck, as salivary glands are very sensitive to radiation. Rapidly progressive dental caries and periodontal disease may ensue and this condition requires the concurrent, intensive application of preventive measures. Apart from treating any basic cause, artificial saliva can be used, but many sufferers find that the frequent sipping of iced water gives the best relief (See Chapter 10). Spicy foods should be avoided, however chewing sugar-free gum may provide relief.

There are some conditions arising elsewhere in the body that can have a visible effect within the mouth, such as pregnancy, anaemia and HIV and AIDS. These also need professional advice and help.

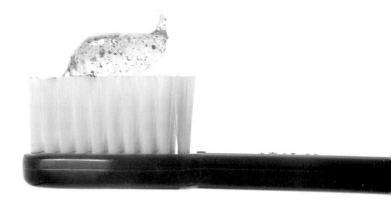

CHAPTER 9.

Advice for children under five

Key points

- Parents should supervise or assist with brushing until children can do it effectively, usually by the age of seven years.
Evidence Base C

- Low-fluoride toothpastes provide only limited anticaries benefit.
Evidence Base A

- A child's normal fluid intake should ideally be plain water or milk.
Evidence Base C

- Food and drinks that do predispose to caries should be limited to main meal times.
Evidence Base B

Toothbrushing

Regular, twice daily, toothbrushing with a fluoride toothpaste can be introduced as soon as practicable after the appearance of the first teeth. However, in the Republic of Ireland, because of widespread water fluoridation, the advice is to brush using a non-fluoride toothpaste up to two years of age and a fluoride containing toothpaste thereafter. A small, soft toothbrush should be used, with just a smear of toothpaste covering initially no more than three-quarters of the brush, increasing from the age of about three years, to a pea-sized amount for children under seven years. A gentle and systematic approach should be used with the aim of cleaning the outside, inside and biting surfaces of all teeth, including the back ones when they appear, usually between one and two years of age. Children should be encouraged to spit out any excess toothpaste after brushing but not to rinse the mouth with water. Younger children are often quite happy to brush their own teeth, but lack the manual dexterity to do so efficiently. Monitoring toothpaste use before seven years of age is also important. Parents should supervise or assist with brushing until the children can do it effectively, usually by the age of seven years. However, some children need supervision beyond this age.

Using a mouthwash that contains fluoride can help prevent dental caries and may provide an additional benefit, however parents should be advised that mouthrinses are not suitable for routine use by children under 6 years of age as they could swallow them accidentally, and many mouthwashes contain alcohol. If they are used on professional advice alcohol-free fluoride mouthwashes are preferred and should not be used directly after brushing. It is also best not to eat or drink for 30 minutes after using a mouthwash.

While a fluoride toothpaste is recommended, low fluoride toothpastes provide only limited anticaries benefit, so for children aged up to three years, toothpaste containing no less than 1,000 ppm fluoride should be used. Children aged from three to six years should use toothpaste containing 1,350-1,500 ppm. However, care must be taken to ensure that younger children do not eat or lick toothpaste from the tube or swallow excessive amounts from the brush (see Chapter 2).

Drinks

Parents and carers of infants should be specifically warned against the practice of allowing prolonged drinking from a bottle, valve-type feeder or any other type of lidded feeder cup of any sugars-sweetened drink, including carbonated drinks, fruit-based juices, squash, natural fruit juice or sweetened tea/coffee. The prolonged contact time between the sugar in the drink and the teeth is well recognised as a cause of rapidly progressive decay, usually of the upper front teeth, resulting in a condition, previously referred to as "nursing bottle caries", but now termed "early childhood caries" (Fig. 9.1). Breast milk, formula and cow's milk all contain the natural sugar lactose and an established pattern of prolonged feeding times can increase the risk of caries. If children are left for any length of time with a bottle, it must only contain water.

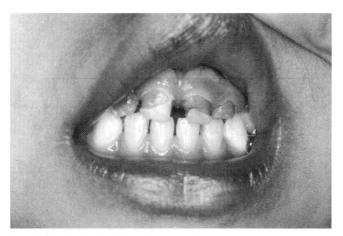

Fig. 9.1   Early childhood caries, better known as 'bottle caries'.

The risk from this practice is increased if the bottle is used to comfort the child, especially at bedtime or when in a cot or pushchair. A bottle should not be used for anything other than milk or water. It is best for parents to move on from a lidded beaker to drinking from a cup as soon as the child is ready. Children should begin moving off the bottle and on to a feeder cup at six months. Bottles should be given up completely by the age of one. There's no need for a child to use a sippy cup. These are similar to a bottle, in that they require the child to suck to make them work. Non-spill (valved) cups are not recommended as they encourage longer drinking times. Lidded free-flow cups are preferable so that the baby learns to sip. If sugars-sweetened drinks are given to younger children, they should be very well diluted, taken preferably at meal times only and drinking times should be kept short. An open cup or beaker should be used, never a bottle. Parents and careers should be aware however, that the sugar content of some flavoured bottled mineral waters can be as high as 10% and the precautions given above for sugars-sweetened drinks should be followed. A child's normal fluid intake should ideally be plain water or milk. Fizzy drinks and fruit juices are acidic and can cause erosion (see Chapter 6) so they should not be given to babies. Fruit smoothies, a blend of fruit and fruit juices have become popular in many countries and are perceived as a healthy drink for children, however they are acidic and frequent consumption can lead to both erosion and caries.

Breast milk is the best form of nutrition for infants. When breastfeeding is not possible cow's milk formulas are the preferred option. Follow-on milks should not be given before 6 months of age and may not be necessary for the majority of children. For infants and children who have an allergy to cow's milk, they should continue on hydrolysed protein infant formulas or soya infant formulas until they are two years old. Hydrolysed protein infant formulas are better nutritionally than those based on soya and infants with an allergy to cow's milk may also have an allergy to soya formula. These infant formulas contain sugars that can cause tooth decay, so it will be particularly important to be careful about caring for the baby's teeth once they start coming through. For infants with severe cow's milk allergy, extensively hydrolysed formulae such as Nutramigen are advised, however they contain glucose syrup and can increase the risk of caries. Parents who have been advised by their GP or other health professional to feed their baby soya-based or hydrolysed protein infant formulas should continue to do so. Feeding times should be kept as short as practical and the advice on toothbrushing and diet should be rigorously followed. The child's dentist should be told of the use of such formulae and additional precautions may be advised.

Teething

It can help to give a teething baby something hard to chew on, such as a teething ring, a crust of bread or breadstick, or a peeled carrot. However, it is important to avoid rusks because almost all contain some sugar; constant chewing and sucking on sugary things can cause tooth decay even if a baby has only one or two teeth. For babies over four months of age, sugar-free teething gel can be rubbed on the gum. The teething gel should not contain salicylate salts. Sugar-free baby paracetamol or ibuprofen preparations may also be used, following the instructions on the bottle for the child's age.

An approximate guide to the different stages of teething is:

- **bottom front teeth (incisors)** – these are the first to come through, at around six to seven months

- **top front teeth (incisors)** – these come through at around six to eight months

- **first molars (back teeth)** – these come through at around 12-16 months

- **canines (towards the back of the mouth)** – these come through at around 12-20 months

- **second molars** – these come through at around 20-30 months

Most children will have all of their milk teeth by the time they are two and a half years old.

Weaning

Parents should be advised to avoid giving sweet things, from the time they start their baby on foods and drinks other than milk and to try to encourage savoury tastes. They should try to avoid giving drinks containing artificial sweeteners, such as saccharin or aspartame. If such drinks are given, they should be diluted with at least 10 parts water to 1 part concentrate. Honey is a mixture of glucose, fructose and sucrose and can cause the same problems as table sugar. Honey should not be given until the age of one year, even for easing coughs. Very occasionally it can contain a type of bacteria which can produce toxins in the baby's intestines and can cause a very serious illness (infant botulism). Foods and drinks that do predispose to caries should be limited to main meal times and sugar-sweetened foods and drinks should not be consumed more than four times per day. Under no circumstances should soothers be dipped into sweetened foods (honey, jam, sugar etc.).

Dental visiting

Children should be taken to the dentist as soon as practicable, and certainly by the time their first teeth appear and then as often as the dentist advises.

Fluoride varnish for children

The Department of Health in England advises that all children over the age of 3 years should have a fluoride varnish professionally applied to the teeth every 6 months or more frequently for children at greater risk of dental caries[1].

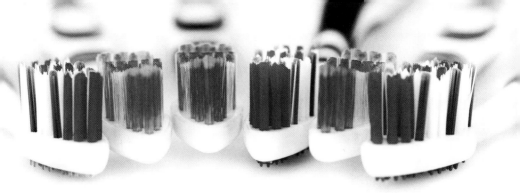

CHAPTER 10

Advice for denture wearers and older people

Key points

- Everyone, including those with full dentures, should have regular oral examinations.
  Evidence Base B

- Dentures should be removed and cleaned every night and should be replaced when damaged, ill-fitting or worn out.
  Evidence Base B

Denture wearers

While the number of denture wearers, especially full dentures, has steadily declined, it is estimated that by 2018, around 5% of the adult population will be edentulous and need full dentures (approximately two million people in the UK); a combination of natural teeth and dentures will still be as common as ever for the next 20 years. Demographic changes suggest an increasing proportion of these will be elderly people and living either alone, possibly receiving community care, or in residential care or nursing care homes. The dental state of people in residential care is often poor, because help needed with oral hygiene may not be available. It is important that the wearers of full or partial dentures, and especially their carers, understand the need for particular care if the health of their mouths and any remaining teeth are to be safeguarded.

Denture cleaning

Routine care should include cleaning of the dentures after every meal and before going to bed. This is necessary to remove the biofilm, bacteria and fungi that accumulate on dentures, especially the fitting surfaces and adherent food debris. Ideally all dentures should be removed before sleeping to allow the soft tissues of the mouth to recover from the denture-bearing load and to remove the risk of injury or Candida infection (see Chapter 8).

Where this is not practical, they should be removed for at least several hours during the day. Denture cleaning should always be done outside the mouth using a small, soft brush and a denture cleaning liquid, paste or liquid soap to clean all denture surfaces before rinsing thoroughly with cold water. Dentures should never be placed in boiling or hot water. While soaking overnight is generally unnecessary, dentures should not be allowed to dry out as they can warp and may be placed in fresh cold tap water or if preferred a proprietary denture soaking solution. Many of these soaking solutions contain hypochlorite, which is bactericidal and helps to break down the organic matrix of adherent plaque that forms on the dentures, but can cause bleaching of denture plastic if dentures are soaked for long periods or in hot water. Hypochlorite is not suitable for prolonged soaking of metal-based dentures for which special soaking solutions containing alkaline peroxide are available. After soaking in proprietary solutions the dentures should be brushed and rinsed with cold water before being inserted. With all cleaning and soaking agents, manufacturer's instructions should be carefully followed. It should be stressed that soaking alone will not clean dentures and thorough brushing before soaking is essential. Any natural teeth should be brushed twice daily with a fluoride toothpaste. The roof of the mouth, the gum ridges and tongue should be gently cleaned daily with a soft brush to remove any food particles and plaque.

Dentures, whether full or partial, do not last indefinitely. The ridges progressively change shape and the edges of the dentures can then begin to irritate the surrounding mucosa. This may cause the dentures to become loose or painful to wear. Even if they remain comfortable, the plastic teeth on the dentures wear down, causing the vertical height between nose and chin to be reduced and the lips to fall in. Often, dentures can be improved by relining the fitting surface, but sometimes older people do not take well to completely new dentures. However, if badly worn, broken or ill-fitting they should be replaced. Because of these considerations, it is advised that denture wearers have their mouths and dentures examined at least every year. The dentures should be examined for the accuracy of fit, any damage and for staining or calculus deposits, which should be removed. As the loss of a denture may cause great distress, especially for older people, dentists making dentures should be asked to include an embedded identification name.

Root caries

An increasing number of elderly people are retaining some or all of their natural teeth. Since many will have periodontal disease with gum recession caries may develop on the exposed root surfaces. This is a common problem, made worse by reduced salivary flow and difficulty in maintaining good plaque control, especially round lower anterior teeth. Treating root caries can be difficult, especially in lower anterior teeth, but poor oral hygiene, possibly aggravated by ill-fitting partial dentures and periodontal disease, in an elderly person in poor health, can result in a major clinical problem. This is potentially an issue for people living in residential care if no oral care plan is in place or is poorly executed. For home care, careful and effective toothbrushing with a high concentration fluoride toothpaste is recommended, together with regular dental check-ups. If teeth are sensitive to hot and cold drinks, the use of a fluoride-containing "sensitive toothpaste" can give relief. However, if discomfort persists, then dental advice should be sought. Fluoride varnish application is an effective aid to caries prevention and can reduce sensitivity, as can topical chlorhexidine varnish, but both require professional application. The use of interdental brushes, especially for cleaning between the lower anterior teeth can be beneficial, but again dental advice should be sought.

Apart from problems related to teeth, gums and dentures, elderly people are more prone to dry mouth (xerostomia), possibly linked to their greater use of multiple medications, and Candida infections of the mouth. This is a distressing and common problem and many sufferers try to stimulate salivary flow by sucking sweets or pastilles or get relief by frequently sipping drinks. However, if these contain sugars they will greatly increase the risk of dental caries. Fortunately an increasing range of sugar-free sweets and mints are available and should be recommended. While artificial saliva substitutes, in the form of sprays or rinses, are available and can give short-term relief, care should be taken to identify those containing animal extracts, which will be unacceptable to some people. Often, frequent sipping of cold water provides the most practical relief. Finally, it must be remembered that the majority of oral cancers occur in the over 60s and swellings or oral ulceration lasting more than three weeks should have immediate professional attention (see Chapter 7).

Oral/dental care of elderly people, especially those in residential care homes, is increasingly a cause for concern. Oral health education for community care, residential and nursing care workers should be a part of their training and should be coordinated with local dental services. An oral care plan should be a required element for all care plans.

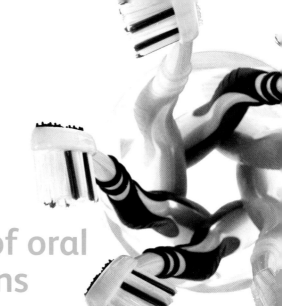

CHAPTER 11:

Frequency of oral examinations

Key points

- There is no evidence that 6-monthly recalls are the optimum frequency.
  Evidence Base C

- Recall intervals should extend from 3 months up to 12 months for under 18 year-olds and up to 24 months for adults.
  Evidence Base C

- The period between examinations should be determined on dental advice and reflect the individual risk of oral disease as well as medical, physical and social factors.
  Evidence Base C

Who needs routine examinations?

While it is accepted that oral examinations at appropriate intervals are of value in maintaining oral health, there is little evidence to support a specific interval or to quantify the benefit. Neither is there evidence that six-monthly recall intervals are the optimum frequency [48]. There are now very many children and adults with little or no dental disease for whom frequent attendance is inappropriate. However, in some areas and among some social groups, the level of oral disease remains high while frequency of attendance is low. The maintenance of periodontal health depends upon effective, daily personal plaque control. Regular professional care may be required at intervals depending on the needs of the individual. With respect to decay, once a definite cavity is present, it cannot be remineralised, but the tooth can be restored and the importance of early detection and appropriate treatment makes dental attendance advisable. Other disorders can occur in the mouth which are unrelated to the presence of natural teeth and which may be life-threatening, for example oral cancers (see Chapter 7).

In October 2004 The UK National Institute for Clinical Excellence published guidance on recall attendance [49]. This states that:

- The shortest interval between oral health reviews for all patients should be 3 months. The longest interval between oral health reviews for patients younger than 18 years should be 12 months.

- The longest interval between oral health reviews for patients aged 18 years and older should be 24 months.

- Recall intervals for patients who have repeatedly demonstrated that they can maintain oral health and who are not considered to be at risk of disease or consequences of oral disease, may be extended over time up to an interval of 24 months. Intervals of longer than 24 months are undesirable because they could diminish the relationship between dentist and patient and people's lifestyles may change during such a period.

- The maximum period of 24 months may be appropriate for adults with no evidence of active dental disease, who are in good general health and do not use tobacco and have low and infrequent sugar and alcohol consumption. Children may need to be seen more frequently, as may those who are at increased risk of oral disease because of smoking, medical, physical or social factors, or for whom dental treatment presents difficulties because of their medical or physical condition. A risk assessment should be made at each recall visit and an appropriate period advised for the next recall. Attendance will enable the health of the whole mouth to be monitored and appropriate dental health advice and early treatment to be provided when needed.

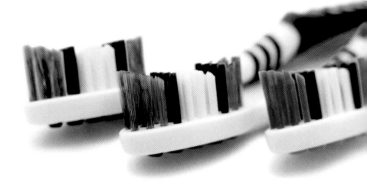

CHAPTER 12:
First aid for traumatised front teeth

Key points

- Professionally made mouthguards should be worn during sporting activities.
  Evidence Base C

- If teeth are fractured, seek immediate dental help and avoid hot or cold liquids and foods.
  Evidence Base C

It is estimated that about 10% of the population have at least one permanent incisor tooth affected by trauma by the age of 15 years and that many remain untreated. These injuries range from the minor, where the teeth can be restored easily by a dentist to cases when one or more whole teeth are knocked out.

The following advice can be given:

- Professionally made mouthguards should be worn during sporting activities. While self-fitted ones are available from many sports shops they can be difficult to accurately mould to the teeth and can become loose and cause choking whilst in use.
- If teeth are fractured, seek immediate dental help and avoid hot or cold liquids and foods.
- If a permanent tooth is knocked out and found, immediate re-implantation can be attempted. The tooth should be held by the crown and contact with the root should be avoided. Any contamination should be gently removed by rinsing with milk or tap water, but no attempt should be made to physically clean or disinfect the tooth. The tooth should be supported by biting on a clean handkerchief or tissue until seen by a dentist. Re-implantation should not be attempted for primary teeth, or if there is any doubt concerning the medical history of the individual.
- If re-implantation is not attempted, the tooth should be placed in a container of saliva, cold milk or even contact lens soaking solution and taken to a dentist.
- Bleeding should be controlled by biting on a clean handkerchief or tissue for 20 minutes.
- Delay in seeking advice can result in the loss of teeth, which could be saved. Where teeth are knocked out, over time the movement of adjacent teeth could narrow the space and make the provision of false teeth more difficult.

Further Reading

Beirne P V, Clarkson J E, Worthington H V. Recall intervals for oral health in primary care patients. *Cochrane Database of Systematic Reviews* 2007, Issue 4. Art. No.: CD004346. DOI: 10.1002/14651858.CD004346.pub3.

Blinkhorn A. Oral health education. In Seward H M, Rothwell P S (eds) *Oral health promotion with Teamwork.* Sheffield: Teamwork Publications, 1997.

British Fluoridation Society. *One in a Million.* Manchester: British Fluoridation Society, 3rd ed. 2012.

Bulletin of the World Health Organisation Volume 83, Number 9, September 2005, 641-720, including 'Diet and nutrition in oral health' by Moynihan P J and 'Oral disease prevention and health promotion' by Watt R G.

Clarkson J, Harrison J E, Ismail A I, Needleman I, Worthington H. *Evidence Based Dentistry for Effective Practice.* London: Martin Dunitz, 2003.

Davies R M, Davies G M, Ellwood R P. Prevention. Part 4: Toothbrushing: what advice should be given to patients? *Br Dent* J 2003; **195**: 135-141.

Daly B, Watt R G, Batchelor P, Treasure E T. *Essential Dental Public Health.* Oxford: OUP; 2013.

Department of Health. *Weaning and The Weaning Diet.* Report of the Working Group on the Weaning Diet of the Committee on Medical Aspects of Food Policy [COMA]. London: HMSO, 1994.

Department of Health. *Choosing Better Oral Health: An Oral Health Plan for England.* London: Department of Health, 2005.

Fejerskov O & Edwina Kidd E A (eds). *Dental Caries: The Disease And Its Clinical Management.* 2nd ed. London: Wiley-Blackwell, 2008.

Griffiths J and Boyle S. *Holistic Oral Care: A Guide for Health Professionals.* London: Stephen Hancocks Limited, 2005.

Health Technology and Assessment NHS R & D HTA Programme report on the clinical effectiveness and cost-effectiveness of routine dental checks: a systematic review and economic evaluation by, Davenport C, Elley K, Salas C, Talyor-Weetman C L, Fry-Smith A, Bryan S, Taylor R. Executive Summary, *Health Technology Assessment* 2003; Vol 7: No 7.

Holbrook W P, Arnadottir I B. Prevention. Part 3. Prevention of tooth wear. *Br Dent* J 2003; **195**: 75-81.

Jenkins W M M, Heasnam P A. The prevention and control of periodontal disease. In Murray J J, Nunn J H, Steele J G (eds). *The Prevention of Oral Disease.* 4th edn, pp. 123-144. Oxford: Oxford Medical Publications, 2003.

Kay E J and Tinsley S R. *Communication and the Dental Team.* London: Stephen Hancocks Limited, 2004.

Kent G, Croucher R. *Achieving Oral Health: the social context of dental care.* Oxford: Wright, 1998.

Marinho V C C, Higgins J P T, Logan S, Sheiham A. Fluoride toothpastes for preventing dental caries in children and adolescents. *Cochrane Database of Systematic Reviews* 2003; Issue 1. Art No,: CD002278. DOI: 10.1002/14651858. CD002278

Moynihan P J. Dietary advice in dental practice. *Br Dent* J 2002; **193**: 563-568.

Moynihan P J. Diet and dental caries. In Murray J J, Nunn J H, Steele J G (eds). *The Prevention of Oral Disease.* 4th edn, pp. 10-34. Oxford: Oxford Medical Publications, 2003.

Murray J J, Rugg-Gunn A, Jenkins G N. *Fluorides in caries prevention.* 3rd edn. Oxford: Butterworth-Heinemann, 1991.

Nuttal N, Steele J, Nunn J G *et al. A Guide to the UK Adult Dental Health Survey 1998.* London: BDJ Books, 2001.

Public Health England, *Water fluoridation: health monitoring report for England 2014*, www.gov.uk/government/publications/water-fluoridation-health-monitoring-report-for-england-2014.

Rugg-Gunn A, Nunn J H. *Nutrition, Diet and Oral Health.* Oxford: Oxford University Press, 1999.

Sheiham A. Dietary effects on dental diseases. *Public Health Nutrition* 2001; 4(2b): 569-591.

Sutcliffe P. Oral cleanliness and dental caries. In Murray J J (ed). *The Prevention of Dental Disease.* 3rd edn, pp. 68-77. Oxford: Oxford Medical Publications, 1996.

Steele J, Walls A. Prevention in the ageing population. In Murray J J, Nunn J H, Steele J G (eds). *The Prevention of Oral Disease.* 4th edn, pp. 190-207. Oxford: Oxford Medical Publications, 2003.

Stillman-Lowe C R. *Oral Health Education: What lessons have we learned?* Oral Health Report 2008; vol 2: 9-13.

Stillman-Lowe CR and Levine R S. *Diet and dental caries.* Oral Health Report 2007; issue 2: 6-12.

Ten Cate J M, Imfeld T (eds). Etiology, mechanism and implications of dental erosion. *European J Oral Sci* 1996; **104**: (2, Pt.2).

Watt R G, McGlone P, Kay E J. Prevention. Part 2: Dietary advice in the dental surgery. *Br Dent J* 2003; **195**: 27-31.

Watt R G, Steele J G, Treasure E T, White D A, Pitts N B & Murray J J. Adult Dental Health Survey 2009: implications of findings for clinical practice and oral health policy. *Br Dent J* 2013; 214: 71-75.

References

1. Public Health England. *Delivering better oral health: An evidence-based toolkit for prevention.* London: Public Health England, 2014.
2. World Health Organization. *The Ottawa Charter for Health Promotion.* Geneva: WHO, 1986.
3. Sheiham A, Watt RG. *The common risk factor approach: a rational basis for promoting oral health.* Community Dent Oral Epidemiol. 2000 Dec;28(6):399-406.
4. Watt RG, Sheiham A *Integrating the common risk factor approach into a social determinants framework.* Community Dent Oral Epidemiol. 2012 Aug;40(4):289-96.
5. Sprod A J, Anderson A, Treasure E T. *Effective oral health promotion: Literature review.* Technical Report 20. Cardiff: Health Promotion Wales, 1996.
6. Kay E J, Locker D. *Effectiveness of oral health promotion: a review.* London: Health Education Authority, 1997.
7. National Institute for Health and Care Excellence. *Behaviour change: individual approaches* (NICE public health guidance 49). London: NICE, 2014.
8. Mason P and Butler C C. *Health Behavior Change: A Guide for Practitioners.* London: Elsevier, 2010.
9. Ramseier C A and Suvan JE (eds). *Health Behavior Change in the Dental Practice.* Iowa: Wiley-Blackwell, 2010.
10. http://www.motivationalinterview.org.
11. Bagramian RA, Garcia-Godoy F, Volpe AR. *The global increase in dental caries. A pending public health crisis.* Am J Dent. 2009 Feb;22(1):3-8. Review.
12. http://www.nwph.net/dentalhealth/survey-results5.aspx?id=1.
13. http://www.cardiff.ac.uk/dentl/research/themes/appliedclinicalresearch/epidemiology/oralhealth/index.html.
14. http://www.scottishdental.org/index.aspx?o=2153&record=416.
15. http://www.dohc.ie/publications/coral.html.
16. Pitts N B, Pine C, Burnside G, Craven R. *Inequalities in dental health in the North-West of England.* Community Dent Health 2003; 20: 53–54.
17. Walsh T, Worthington HV, Glenny AM, Appelbe P, Marinho VC, Shi X. *Fluoride toothpastes of different concentrations for preventing dental caries in children and adolescents.* Cochrane Database Syst Rev. 2010 Jan 20;(1):CD007868. doi: 10.1002/14651858.CD007868.pub2.
18. https://www.york.ac.uk/inst/crd/fluorid.htm.
19. Parnell C, Whelton H, O'Mullane D. *Water fluoridation.* Eur Arch Paediatr Dent. 2009 Sep;10(3):141-8.
20. Marinho VC *Cochrane reviews of randomized trials of fluoride therapies for preventing dental caries.* Eur Arch Paediatr Dent. 2009 Sep;10(3):183-91.
21. Marinho VC, Worthington HV, Walsh T, Clarkson JE. *Fluoride varnishes for preventing dental caries in children and adolescents.* Cochrane Database Syst Rev. 2013 Jul 11;7:CD002279. doi: 10.1002/14651858. CD002279.pub2.
22. Marinho VC, Higgins JP, Logan S, Sheiham A. *Fluoride mouthrinses for preventing dental caries in children and adolescents.* Cochrane Database Syst Rev. 2003;(3):CD002284. doi: 10.1002/14651858.CD002284.

23. Tubert-Jeannin S. *et al. Fluoride supplements (tablets, drops, lozenges or chewing gums) for preventing dental caries in children.* Cochrane database Syst Rev. 2011 Dec 7;(12):CD007592. doi: 10.1002/14651858.CD007592.pub2.

24. Bánóczy J, Rugg-Gunn A, Woodward M. *Milk fluoridation for the prevention of dental caries.* Acta Med Acad. 2013 Nov;42(2):156-67. doi:10.5644/ama2006-124.83.

25. Yeung A, Hitchings JL, Macfarlane TV, Threlfall A, Tickle M, Glenny A. *Fluoridated milk for preventing dental caries.* Cochrane Database of Systematic Reviews 2005, Issue 3. Art. No.: CD003876. doi: 10.1002/14651858.CD003876.pub2

26. Wong MC, Glenny AM, Tsang BW, Lo EC, Worthington HV, Marinho VC *Topical fluoride as a cause of dental fluorosis in children.* Cochrane Database Syst Rev. 2010 Jan 20;(1):CD007693. doi: 10.1002/14651858. CD007693.pub2.

27. Ahovuo-Saloranta A, Forss H, Walsh T, Hiiri A, Nordblad A, Mäkelä M, Worthington HV. *Sealants for preventing dental decay in the permanent teeth.* Cochrane Database Syst Rev. 2013 Mar 28;3:CD001830. doi: 10.1002/14651858.CD001830.pub4.

28. Department of Health. *Dietary sugars and human disease - Report of the Committee on Medical Aspects of Food Policy* [COMA]. London: HMSO, 1989.

29. https://www.gov.uk/government/publications/national-diet-and-nutrition-survey-results-from-years-1-to-4-combined-of-the-rolling-programme-for-2008-and-2009-to-2011-and-2012.

30. Maguire A, Rugg-Gunn A J. *Xylitol and caries prevention – is it a magic bullet?* Br Dent J 2003; 194: 429–438.

31. World Health Organisation. *Diet, Nutrition and the Prevention of Chronic Diseases.* Report of a Joint WHO/FAO Expert Consultation. Geneva: World Health Organisation, 2003.

32. Levine R S. *Caries experience and bedtime consumption of sugar-sweetened foods and drinks – a survey of 600 children.* Community Dent Health 2001; 18: 228–231.

33. Grossi SG, Genco RJ. *Periodontal disease and diabetes mellitus: A two-way relationship.* Ann Periodontol 1998; 3: 51-61.

34. Chapple ILC & Genco RJ. *Diabetes and periodontal diseases: consensus report of the Joint EFP/AAP Workshop on Periodontitis and Systemic Diseases.* J Clin Periodontol 2013; 40 (Suppl. 14): S106–S112 and J Periodontol 2013; 84 (4 Suppl.): S106-S112 .

35. Levine R S. *Obesity, diabetes and periodontitis--a triangular relationship?* Br Dent J. 2013 Jul;215(1):35-9.

36. Kinane DF, Chestnutt IG. *Smoking and periodontal disease.* Crit Rev Oral Biol Med. 2000;11(3):356-65.

37. Poklepovic T, Worthington HV, Johnson TM, Sambunjak D, Imai P, Clarkson JE, Tugwell P. *Interdental brushing for the prevention and control of periodontal diseases and dental caries in adults.* Cochrane Database Syst Rev. 2013 Dec 18;12:CD009857. doi: 10.1002/14651858.CD009857.pub2.

38. Robinson P G, Deacon S A, Deery C, Heanue M, Walmsley A D, Worthington H V, Glenny A M, Shaw W C. *Manual versus powered toothbrushing for oral health.* Cochrane Data- base of Systematic Reviews 2005, Issue 2. Art. No.: CD002281.

doi: 10.1002/14651858.

39. Dugmore CR, Rock WP. *A multifactorial analysis of factors associated with dental erosion.* Br Dent J. 2004 Mar 13;196(5):283-6.

40. Young A, Amaechi BT, Dugmore C, Holbrook P, Nunn J, Schiffner U, Lussi A, Ganss C. *Current erosion indices--flawed or valid?* Summary. Clin Oral Investig. 2008 Mar;12 Suppl 1:S59-63.

41. Kreulen C.M. Van't Spijker A. Rodriguez J.M. Bronkhorst E.M. Creugers N.H.J. Bartlett D.W. *Systematic Review of the Prevalence of Tooth Wear in Children and Adolescents.* Caries Res 2010;44:151–159.

42. http://www.cancerresearchuk.org/cancer-info/cancerstats.

43. Radoï L, Luce D. *A review of risk factors for oral cavity cancer: the importance of a standardized case definition.* Community Dent Oral Epidemiol. 2013;41(2):97-109.

44. http://www.cancerresearchuk.org/cancer-info/cancerstats/types/oral/riskfactors/.

45. Werner CW, Seymour RA. *Are alcohol containing mouthwashes safe?* Br Dent J. 2009 Nov 28;207(10):E19.

46. D'Souza G & Dempsey A. *The role of HPV in head and neck cancer and review of the HPV vaccine.* Preventive Medicine 2011; 53:Sup.1 S5–S1

47. Stanley M Perspective: *Vaccinate boys too.* Nature 2012;488, S10

48. Riley P, Worthington HV, Clarkson JE, Beirne PV. *Recall intervals for oral health in primary care patients.* Cochrane Database Syst Rev. 2013 Dec 19;12:CD004346. doi: 10.1002/14651858.CD004346.pub4.

49. National Institute for Clinical Excellence. Clinical Guideline 19. *Dental recall: recall interval between routine dental examinations.* London: NICE, 2004.

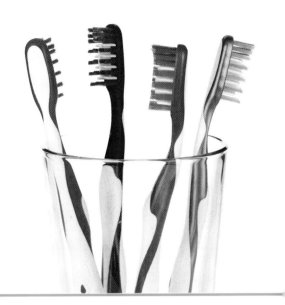

Appendices

Appendix 1: Smoking cessation for the dental team

Appendix 2: Guidelines for healthy eating

Appendix 3: Eruption dates for teeth

Appendix 4: Useful websites

Appendix 5: List of expert advisers

Appendix 1

Smoking cessation for the dental team

Key points

- The dental team should promote smoking cessation among their patients. Evidence Base A

Smoking and the use of smokeless tobacco are a major public health problem in England. Each year more than 70,000 people die prematurely of tobacco-related diseases. Tobacco use is a major cause of health inequalities as rates of smoking remain high among socially disadvantaged groups. Tobacco use is also a major threat to oral health. Oral cancer and periodontal diseases are directly caused by tobacco. Nearly 1,900 people die from oral cancer each year in England and rates are increasing, especially among younger people. Reducing tobacco use across the population is therefore a major priority for Public Health England. Dental teams are in an ideal position to provide very brief advice to tobacco users.

Public Health England has therefore published a second edition of *Smokefree and Smiling: Helping dental patients to quit tobacco* in 2014. This document provides updated guidance for dental teams, commissioners and educators on how they can contribute to reducing rates of tobacco use, and highlights resources available to support them.

The report's key recommendations are:

1. People who use tobacco should receive advice to stop and be offered support to do so with a referral to their local stop smoking service.

2. Dental schools, postgraduate deaneries and other providers and commissioners of dental teaching should ensure that tobacco cessation training is available and meets national standards.

3. Dental teams are routinely proactive in engaging users of tobacco.

4. Commissioning bodies implement appropriate measures that support the above recommendations.

Recommendation 1

People who use tobacco should receive advice to stop and be offered support to do so with a referral to their local stop smoking service.

The National Centre for Smoking Cessation and Training (NCSCT) has developed a simple form of advice designed to be used opportunistically in less than 30 seconds in almost any consultation with a tobacco user. It is called very brief advice (VBA).

In the vast majority of cases, dental teams will only be involved in delivering VBA to tobacco users. Using the following pathway will increase the chance of a successful quit attempt and reduce time of delivery. It has three elements:

1. Establishing and recording smoking status (ASK)
2. Advising on the personal benefits of quitting (ADVISE)
3. Offering help (ACT)

A large study of advice given by GPs across England, found that smokers were almost twice as likely to try to stop when they received an offer of help rather than just advice to stop. When compared with no advice to smokers, recommending treatment or support via VBA increased the odds of quitting by 68% and 217% respectively.

Ask

All patients should have their tobacco use (current/ex/never used) established and checked at least once a year. The member of the dental team who elicits this information should update it in the patient's clinical notes.

Advise

Having established that people are smokers, the traditional approach has been to warn them of the dangers and advise them to stop. This is deliberately left out of VBA for two reasons:

1. It can immediately create a defensive reaction and raise anxiety levels
2. It takes time and can generate a conversation about their tobacco use, which is more appropriate during a dedicated stop smoking consultation

There is no need to ask how long someone has used tobacco, how much they use, or even what they use (cigarettes, shisha, cigars, chewing tobacco or paan). Stopping use will be beneficial in every case and the details of this are better saved for the stop smoking consultation. The best way of assessing a smoker's motivation to stop is simply to ask, *"Do you want to stop smoking/ chewing tobacco?"*

VBA involves a simple statement advising that the best way to stop is with a combination of support and treatment, which can significantly increase the chance of stopping.

Act

All smokers receive advice about the value of attending their local stop smoking services for specialised help. Those who are interested and motivated to stop receive a referral to these services.

For some people, it might not be the right time to stop. For those not interested in stopping, a simple "that is fine but help will always be available, let me know if you change your mind" works best.

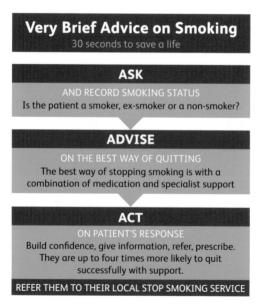

Fig. A1.

Recommendation 3

Dental teams are proactive in engaging users of tobacco.

Local stop smoking services have helped many thousands of people to successfully stop using tobacco. In 2011- 12 over 400,000 people (49% of attendees) stopped by using these services. Indeed, smokers are up to four times more likely to stop if they attend these services and use medication than if they try to quit on their own without support and medication. As a result, policy guidance to health professionals now emphasises the importance of referring everybody who wants to stop using tobacco to the local stop smoking service for specialist assistance and support.

- The best outcomes occur when smokers who want to stop take-up a referral for specialist support. Timing is crucial: the quicker the contact from a local stop smoking service, the greater the smoker's motivation and interest. Dental patients who say they want to stop and are directed to their local stop smoking services receive the best opportunity to stop smoking. The dental team's role is vital in telling the patient how to contact the local service. It just takes 30 seconds and can give patients the motivation to seek professional help, which increases their chances of quitting.

- Dental teams and the local stop smoking services can work collaboratively in a variety of ways. As a first step it is important all members of a dental team are fully aware of the services offered locally and of how these operate. Arranging a meeting with a representative of a local service can be a useful opportunity for dental teams to learn about the service and the best ways of directing dental patients to it.

- Teams working together provide much more support to people who want to stop smoking. It is important that no matter who makes the referral the patient's progress is assessed and recorded in their clinical notes at each subsequent dental appointment. Many people find it difficult to stop smoking and it is often associated with a range of unpleasant, short-term withdrawal symptoms – some, such as ulcers, directly affect the oral cavity. Reassurance and advice from dental teams can help patients deal more effectively with these problems, and increase their chances of quitting successfully.

- Advice and support should only be delivered by staff trained to the current NCSCT training standard. Preferably, they should be fully NCSCT certified, having passed the knowledge (Stage 1) and practice (Stage 2) assessments. In this case, as with any provider of services, continued commitment to governance and performance monitoring will ensure patients are to be provided with the best available intervention.

Among certain ethnic minority groups, chewing tobacco and/or areca nut (paan) is common. Evidence associates chewing tobacco and other products with oral cancers and other oral pathologies. A recent Cochrane systematic review showed that advice delivered in dental surgeries is effective in helping tobacco chewers to stop. Current NICE guidance on smokeless tobacco users in south Asian communities, recommends dental teams: ask people if they use smokeless tobacco, using the local names of the various products. If necessary, show them a picture of what the products look like (this may be necessary if the person does not speak English well or does not understand the terms used). Inform the patient of the health risks (for example, lung cancer, respiratory illness and periodontal disease) associated with tobacco use and advise them to stop. Refer anybody who wants to quit to the available local specialist tobacco cessation service. Record the outcome in the patient's notes. Use the same VBA (Ask, Advise, Act) method for smokers and smokeless tobacco users.

Appendix 2
Guidelines for a healthy diet

Key point

- Dietary advice for patients given by the dental team should be consistent with general healthy eating guidelines. Evidence Base C

The two keys to a healthy diet are to:

- Eat the right number of calories for how active you are, so that you balance the energy you consume with the energy you lose. Most adults are eating more calories than they need, and should eat fewer calories.
- Eat a wide range of foods to ensure that you're getting a balanced diet and that your body is receiving all the nutrients it needs.

Consumers should aim to:

1. Base their meals on starchy foods, such as bread, cereals, rice, pasta and potatoes, choosing wholegrain varieties whenever possible. Starchy food should make up around one third of the food you eat.
2. Eat lots of fruit and vegetables – aiming for at least five portions of a variety of fruit and vegetables every day.
3. Eat more fish, aiming for two portions a week, including one portion of oily fish.
4. Most people in the UK eat and drink too much sugar. Sugary foods and drinks, including alcoholic drinks, are often high in energy and could contribute to weight gain.
5. Eat less salt. Even if you don't add salt to your food, you may still be eating too much. About three-quarters of the salt we eat is already in the food we buy. Use food labels to help you cut down.
6. Get active and be a healthy weight. Most adults need to lose weight and need to eat fewer calories in order to do this.

7. Drink plenty of water – aim to drink about six to eight glasses (1.2 litres) of water, or other fluids, every day. Drinking too much alcohol can cause problems: women can drink up to two to three units of alcohol a day and men up to three to four units a day, without significant risk to their health.

8. Avoid skipping breakfast – missing meals doesn't help weight loss.

The eatwell plate illustrated below shows the types and proportions of foods that make up a healthy and well balanced diet.

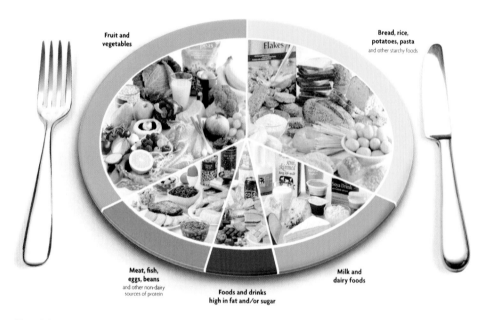

Fig. A2.

Appendix 3
Eruption dates of teeth

Deciduous teeth (months)			
Incisors	canines	1st molars	2nd molars
6-8	12-20	12-16	20-30

Permanent teeth (years)		
	Lower	Upper
1st Incisor	6-7	7-8
2nd Incisor	7-8	8-9
Canine	9-10	11-12
1st premolar	9-12	9-12
2nd premolar	10-12	10-12
1st Molar	6-7	6-7
2nd Molar	10-12	11-13
3rd Molar	17-21	17-21

Appendix 4

Useful evidence-based dentistry websites

- **Centre for Evidence-based Medicine**
  www.cebm.net/

- **Centre for Evidence-based Dentistry**
  www.cebd.org/

- **Cochrane Oral Health Group**
  www.ohg.cochrane.org/

- **NHS Choices**
  www.nhs.uk/Pages/HomePage.aspx

- **NHS Centre for Reviews and Dissemination, University of York**
  www.york.ac.uk/inst/crd/

- **National Institute for Health Research** (NIHR) **Health Technology Assessment Programme**
  www.nets.nihr.ac.uk/programmes/hta

- **National Institute for Health and Care excellence** (NICE)
  www.nice.org.uk/

- **Public Health England**
  www.gov.uk/government/organisations/public-health-england

- **Royal College of Surgeons, Faculty of Dental Surgery**
  www.rcseng.ac.uk/fds/publications-clinical-guidelines/clinical_guidelines

- **Scottish Intercollegiate Guidelines Network** (SIGN)
  www.sign.ac.uk/

- **The Scottish Dental Clinical Effectiveness Programme**
  www.sdcep.org.uk/

Appendix 5
Panel of expert advisors

Professor I L C Chapple
School of Dentistry, University of Birmingham.

Professor S Creanor
Department of Oral Sciences, Peninsula Schools of Medicine and Dentistry, Plymouth University.

Dr V C Marinho
Barts and The London School of Medicine and Dentistry, Queen Mary, University of London.

Professor P J Moynihan
Centre for Oral Health Research, Institute of Health and Society, Newcastle University.

Professor J Nunn
School of Dental Science, University of Dublin.

Professor P M Preshaw
School of Dental Sciences, Newcastle University.

Professor A Sheiham
Department of Epidemiology & Public Health, University College London.

Professor P M Speight
School of Clinical Dentistry, University of Sheffield.

WITHDRAWN
FROM STOCK
LIBR